Controlling My Life?

How to Achieve Positive Mental Health Outcomes for Minority Ethnic Communities from Their Own Perspectives

Controlling My Life?

How to Achieve Positive Mental Health Outcomes for Minority Ethnic Communities from Their Own Perspectives

Dr. Stephen Joseph

With foreword by Professor Frank Keating

Exceller Books

EXCELLER BOOKS
A GLOBAL PRESS

Controlling My Life?

How to Achieve Positive Mental Health Outcomes for Minority Ethnic Communities from Their Own Perspectives

Cover design by Exceller Books using resources from Pixabay.com

ISBN: 978-93-90746-81-1

First published in India in 2021 by Exceller Books

Address: G1, Dream Apartment, Degree College Road, Belgharia, Kolkata, 700056, India

EXCELLER BOOKS
A GLOBAL PRESS

www.excellerbooks.com

Dedication

This book is dedicated to the glory of God in the first instance; the Maker of Heaven and Earth, Omnipotent, Omniscient and Omnipresent, and from whom all life and forms emanate.

Then to the service users who have agreed to share their life experiences with mental health challenges, and their views. They have inspired me to write this book from a PhD thesis, as I owe them a depth of gratitude, and a sense of responsibility to use this book to give them a voice, as the 'unheard', people who have expressed that they have not been listened to in their lived experiences of mental ill health.

Foreword

Racial disparities across all indicators of health and well-being and in particular in mental health have been a longstanding feature of the lived experience of racialised minorities in the United Kingdom. There is well documented evidence that individuals from these groups have more adverse pathways to mental health services, experience the harsher end of treatment and care and therefore have poorer outcomes than their white counterparts. We also know that African and Caribbean communities are disproportionately affected. Anecdotes from service users from these groups indicate that they have to hand over a great deal of control over their lives once they come into contact with mental health services. However, they find it hard to regain that control once they embark on a journey to recovery. As far as I am aware the importance of the issues pertaining to control has not been examined in any great depth. This timely book sheds light on how issues of control are understood by African and Caribbean service users from their perspective. It draws from an original study in the UK and for the first time explores the concept of 'Locus of Control', what this means for African and Caribbean service users and how this impacts their mental health experiences. What is novel about this book is that it documents the voices of service users, something that is seldom addressed in studies on mental health and 'race'. Service users are often written, talked about, and their stories are seldom told in their voices – this book does this! It gives greater insight into how issues of culture, 'race', racism and other social factors affect the lived experiences of service users and points to how this can be used to inform appropriate and responsive mental health care.

This book is divided into three parts: starting with the voices of service users where direct accounts are given of their understanding on issues of control and care; then moving on to conceptual and theoretical issues; and closes with an analysis of the implications for mental health practice and solutions for change. It is a must read for practitioners, students, researchers and policy makers.

Frank Keating

Caveat Emptor

Caveat emptor is a Latin term that means "let the buyer beware" applies to this book

It is not intended to be a run on the mill, conventional, or 'normal' book

It is not aimed to be 'politically correct';

Neither is it intended to be 'academically correct'

It is my attempt to 'tell it like it is' as much as possible, from my experience as a PhD researcher into mental health in ethnic communities in United Kingdom (Joseph, 2018), and a snippet from other countries.

The research originated from what I have observed over many years of my exposure to mental health and challenges relating to disparity and inequality in outcomes in the United Kingdom and overseas. I have also based the focus of this book on the experiences of the Black and Minority Ethnic (BME) peoples, particularly individuals of Caribbean and African origin. Some references are also made to minority groups in other countries, including Australia, where they are commonly referred to as 'Culturally And Linguistically Diverse' (CALD) peoples.

It is my interest to give 'voice' to the people who have kindly volunteered to share their experiences of mental health challenges, and mental health services in the United Kingdom, despite their misgivings about participating in research.

I feel that I owe them this much to enable them to use this as a platform to air their views, as they are considered 'hard to reach communities' in academic parlance.

As a result of this, I have taken the liberty to avoid as much as I can, the purported 'nuanced interpretation' of the views the interviewees have expressed, as is usually required by the academic community. I have, however, added research elements to the book for the benefit of students, health professionals and all stakeholders interested in research, mental health, and minority communities. This includes the background information, principles, conceptualisation, processes, challenges, and reflections on conducting research into the subject communities.

Consequently, this book is divided into the following parts:

Part 1 contains

- A brief introduction of the study that I carried out with the participation of individuals who described themselves as African and Caribbean peoples and have experiences of mental illness, and mental health services, including experience of psychiatric hospital admissions in the United Kingdom.
- The results of the study, and my thoughts on the different areas of the findings.

Part 2 contains

- The background and theoretical issues that guided the study.

Part 3 contains

- The concluding components that explore the application and implications of the findings in this book for peoples of culture worldwide. It also draws on applicability of the challenges, findings, and implications to ethnic, migrant, and indigenous examples from other countries, including Australia.

I deliberately used this method, as I feel that the contents of part one is more important, as the voices of the participants need to be heard, because it has not been the case for many years. There has been a lot of talk about the over-representation of BME peoples in mental health hospitals and services, but many of the information out there have not actually asked the people with experience of the services to share their experiences and opinions in considerable depth. In doing this, I have included as many quotes as possible without making too many interpretations, as I wanted the quotes to have their own voices and speak to the reader.

This is also in the hope that the policy makers and health professionals of all cadres and persuasion will find it useful to gain more insight into the major problems of over-representation and inequality of outcomes of BME peoples in general and A & C peoples in the United Kingdom, as well as its application to other minority cultures, as patients/service users/consumers/clients (as they are referred to), in mental health settings, in comparison to their population percentages and the representation and outcomes of members of the mainstream population. The book will also appeal to the mental health services worldwide where minority ethnic peoples are receiving services, particularly in relation to the use of the mental health Act/Law and other restrictive practices, irrespective of whatever reasons are given for the practices. I also hope that health professionals, policy makers and government entities will be able to apply some of the suggestions made here to address the challenges of mental health outcomes of ethnic minority populations. I have also tried to make the first part of this book readable as much as possible, by doing what I call 'toning down' the jargons that can be found in many academic books in order to ease understanding and user-friendliness.

Why This Book?
Where It All Began

This is an expose on my motivation for writing this book. It contains the origin of my experience as a nursing student, my exposure to mental health during placements, my deliberate decision to focus on this field, my experience with research and how mental health and wellbeing ultimately became my passion.

My first exposure to mental health occurred in my second year of studying Master of Nursing Science in the University of Melbourne when I took a unit in mental health. I was surprised at the rate of mental health challenges and was opportuned to have a discussion with a mental health service user who was a guest lecturer in one of my classes. I subsequently participated in placements at major hospitals in Melbourne where I had the opportunity to 'shadow' psychiatric nurses as a nursing student in my clinical placement days. This was where the thought of becoming a mental health nurse originated, as many of my preceptors and managers gave me positive feedback about what they had observed that I was able to interact positively with many of their patients. Indeed, many of them stated that I was a 'natural'. On completion of my nursing degree, I applied and was successful in gaining employment into a graduate programme in another city in Australia, where I worked as a psychiatric nurse with rotations to several categories of inpatient settings, including adult and older persons (over 65). I also enrolled into the Postgraduate mental health programme with another university.

I experienced a personal challenge in my early experience as a mental health nurse. This was in physically restraining patients who were presumed to be going through psychotic states. These patients were considered potentially violent, and decisions were made within multidisciplinary teams of Doctors, Nurses, Social Workers and other allied health professionals to administer rapid tranquillisation on the clients, ostensibly to 'calm' them down. I also found the experience of managing seclusion, by putting someone in a small room, with a mattress on the concrete floor, Styrofoam cups of water, and observing them every fifteen minutes, as a source of conflict between caring for mental health clients on the one hand while applying physical force on the other. I also noticed the negative impact of this practice on the therapeutic relationship in the subsequent interactions between the nurse and the patient, who continued to be cared for in the acute and community settings. I found it quite intriguing also that many of the patients would relate their experiences during the restraints and seclusion, mentioning the nurses that they found to be rude and violent to them, and their feeling of helplessness. It is also interesting that I used to be the nurse on duty asked to administer the injections on such patients and found that the patients would remind me of some specific details of their experiences.

Out of curiosity, I decided to conduct a study into seclusion as a practice, as part of the research component of my postgraduate mental health programme. I found that there had been concerted efforts in many countries to eliminate the practice (Grigg, 2006; Lafond, 2007; Allen, de Nesnera & Souther, 2009; Hamilton & Love, 2010). In the United States of America (USA), it was reported that by the year 2006, the efforts by the Pennsylvania state to eliminate seclusion in "civil and forensic services" (Smith, et al, 2006:577), resulted in 99.9% rate compared with the 1996 levels (Smith, et al, 2006:577). The researcher's study did not, however, find any evidence to indicate that similar initiatives had been introduced or tried in the United Kingdom at the time leading to my research conducted in 2011. On arriving back to the UK, I was opportuned to gain employment as a community participatory research assistant with St George's University of London (2012 to 2013). The research experience, which involved the evaluation of a project aimed at raising awareness of BME people about mental health in south west London, opportuned me to participate in workshops, record several events and conduct interviews with members of the community. This experience exposed me to the challenges in the profile of BME mental health in the United Kingdom and the mental health services' concern over the overrepresentation, and the high incidence of seclusion and restraint experienced by the BME population and other coercive practices.

I also pondered deeply on the identified challenges of racism, racial discrimination and a high sense of inequality expressed by many BME mental health service users, family members, and close associates in their experiences with mental health services. The literature review I conducted at this time unearthed several research and reports such as 'Breaking the circles of fear' (Keating et al, 2002), and the *Delivering Race Equality* (DRE) (Crisp et al, 2016) had also highlighted issues of racial inequality and institutional racism playing significant roles in the experiences of BME communities in the United Kingdom. I also participated in several community mental health awareness programs in South London, including the 'Healing our Broken Village' in 2013 organised by the Wandsworth Community Empowerment Network (WCEN), in which several academics, representatives of charity organisations and mental health practitioners also highlighted the problems around racism, a lack of understanding of BME peoples, ethnicity, history and cultures by mental health services as paramount factors in the reported negative BME mental health experiences.

Several mentions were also made in these forums regarding BME people feeling that there was a sense of a lack of control in the experiences of the service users, their family members and friends whenever they were admitted to mental health hospitals, and a sense of dissatisfaction with services. As my earlier view as a practitioner who had been participating in some of the practices that involved limitation of service users' control such as seclusion and restraint, these observations in the community events constituted a basis of further concern and discomfort for me. I continued to struggle with the thought around the conflict between limiting people's freedom and sense of control obtained from the provisions of the Mental Health Act, whilst supposedly caring for them in clinical and community mental health settings. While considering these exposures along with my knowledge of mental health, then my interest was also kindled, as I could not help but wonder if such experiences of limited freedom could also become my lot if, per chance, I should experience mental health challenges as a Black male living in the United Kingdom and end up in having to be cared for by the same mental health services. These exposures also impacted on my pre-existing views that the issues of racism and other reports of poor mental health care experiences could have a root in a poor understanding of the ethnicity and cultures of BME peoples by mental health services that merited further investigation. Also, as a member of the BME community of African descent, I felt a sense of responsibility as a health professional and researcher to find out what could be contributing to the societal challenge of having many members of my community in mental health institutions, and the impact on mental illness sufferers, their families and society at large. In addition, as an advocate of evidence-based practice, and as a follow-up to my previous study on seclusion, I felt the need to contribute to knowledge towards an improvement in the observed challenges, promote cultural competency and enhance positive clinical and community mental health practices.

My interest in exploring the tension between care and control as explained here resulted in my quest to undertake a PhD programme. I decided that I needed to provide evidence that can be referred to by the health services and policy makers in order to address the inequality in outcomes of mental health of BME communities in comparison to the mainstream population. I was also interested in exploring my interest in healthcare research, as the seed was sown during my nursing programme in Australia, when I was amongst a group of students and lecturers that carried out an investigation into factors associated with incidents of aggression in a general inpatient setting, which resulted in a Journal publication (Williamson, et al, 2014).

My literature review resulted in identification of Locus of Control, which was a God-sent concept for me, as I found it, with the guidance of my PhD supervisor, to be an appropriate tool that I could use to explore the tension between care and control. Locus of control is defined as the extent to which individuals perceive that they have control over events that impact their lives (Papadopoulos, 2009; Morling & Kitayama, 2008 Cheng et al, 2013).

Table of Contents

Part I

Introduction

Two focus group interview sessions (a total of eight women and six men), and ten one to one interviews (six women and four men) were conducted with African and Caribbean peoples with experience of mental illness, and mental health services in the United Kingdom, including several hospital admissions. They were asked to share their experiences and views on what constitutes control for them, and how this relates to the origin of their mental health challenges, their mental illness experiences, and their experiences with mental health services, in line with research processes as explained in part two. This part of the book contains the results, including details of the topics identified from the interviews. To protect the identity of the study participants, aliases have been used in the results (Griffiths et al, 2011). The extracts from one-to-one interviews are presented as (Name, 1-1) and from focus groups as (Name, FG1 or Name, FG2).

Topics from results –Superordinate and Subordinate

A total of five superordinate topics and several respective subordinate topics have been identified from both the one-to-one and focus group interview sessions in this study following analysis using the Interpretive Phenomenological Analysis (IPA), based on the responses of the study participants to the questions in the interview schedule and focus group guide. As shown in the Table 1 below, the five superordinate topics include: Meaning of control; Level of Control in relation to mental health experience; Role of culture in mental health Locus of Control; Experiences of Care and Control with services; and Suggestions for improving the experiences of African and Caribbean groups with services.

Super ordinate Topics	Subordinate topics
1.Perception of Control-meaning	1.0 Taking important decisions 1.1- On everyday matters 1.2 – Regarding mental health 1.3- Spirituality in taking decisions
2. Perception of Levels of Control in relation to mental health experience	2.0 Levels of control- mental illness triggers 2.0.1 – Stress factors 2.0.2 - Identity challenges 2.1 Different levels of control-services experience 2.1.1 Admission process & hospital experience 2.1.2 Level of control-contradictory post discharge experiences
3.The role of culture in LOC	3.1- Significance of culture in identity and LOC 3.2 Significance of family in culture and LOC 3.3 Perception that their culture was being ignored in respect of diet and other support for self-care in hospitals 3.4 Low perception of African and Caribbean ethnicity and cultures by mental health services
4.Experiences of Care & Control in Mental Health services	4.1 Coercive practices 4.2 Lack of consistent care 4.3 'Earning' discharge 4.4 Personal needs not being met.

5.Suggestions for improving experience for African and Caribbean clients	5.1 Staffing by African and Caribbean, including senior roles/models 5.2 Professionals to show interest in the culture of African and Caribbean people 5.3. Listening to ideas of clients and their family members 5.4 Post discharge support 5.5 Community approaches 5.6 Clients approaches

Table 1: Super Ordinate and Subordinate Topics Emerging From the Results

1| Meaning of Control over One's Life-Taking Important Decisions

As indicated in the methodology section, the semi-structured interview questions administered to the participants in both one-to-one and focus group settings were designed to obtain answers to the research questions. The first set of questions was aimed at seeking an understanding of the LOC perspective of the participants. This was based on the premise that control over one's life is attributable to the extent to which one can take decisions over one's life. It was attempted by asking questions around decision making, in order to untangle the extent to which the participants relied on other people outside of themselves to take important decisions. For example, the first set of questions asked: *How do you take decisions that are important to your life?* This is followed by a prompt: *Do you ask anyone before you take decisions?* In order to further explore their understanding of LOC, participants were also asked to comment and discuss their understanding of being in control of one's life. These set of questions resulted in this superordinate theme of the participants' perspective regarding how decisions are taken by them. Three subordinate topics emerged around decision making; these were taking decisions on everyday issues, deciding on issues regarding mental health, and spirituality. They indicated that their decision making centred around the role of family members and friends on everyday issues of importance which were not mental health related. However, a difference emanated as to whom they consult on issues regarding mental health. Their responses also highlighted the role played by spirituality in consultation with spiritual leaders and reliance on prayers in their decisions. The subtopics raise some factors that are considered in the type of important decisions referred to by most of the participants. It has been indicated within this superordinate theme and the accompanying subordinate topics, that the participants have made a distinction in the types of decisions, by expressing a difference in whom they would consult when they face mental health challenges. The findings in this theme also challenges the general notion in literature regarding decision making by BME groups, to the effect that as belonging to collectivist cultures, they tend to rely on family and friends on matters of importance.

1.1. Decisions on Everyday Matters -The Role of Family Members and Friends

Within this subtheme the participants linked their decision making on everyday important matters to the importance of the role played by members of their family and friends. When they were asked how they made important decisions in their lives, most of the participants responded that they relied on family members and friends before making decisions on issues of importance. One example of this perception is contained in this statement by Kay who stated that she would consult her son first-hand, whom she referred to as her carer, before making important decisions. She also considers her son as 'the important person' in her life, and the person she would make important decisions with:

> *"Well, the first person I would consult is my son because my son has been my carer over many years and has been there with me through all the peaks and troughs of my life. So I would always make really, really important decisions with him and talk to him about it because he's got keys to my front door to come and keep an eye on me at least once a week. So he's the important person in my life."* (Kay, 1-1)

Another example of reliance on family members and the importance of such members in decision making by many of the participants was contained in the statement expressed by Melissa, who stated that her sister was important to her, and that she would 'go to her first' before taking important decisions.

> *"Well my senior sister, who lives in xxx, is very important to me, I'd probably go to her first believe it or not"*

This perception of influence of members of the family in decision making is further exemplified in the level to which many of the participants attribute the presence of family members to their own lives. For example, it was highlighted in Carla's statement regarding her son, as she also added that her decisions were influenced by her son, and whom she 'lived for'*:*

> *"Basically, my son influences my decisions because he's all I've got. He's the person I live for with my grandchildren of course".*

Brian also stated that he relies on his sister to help him making decisions, he also attributed his reliance on her to avoid getting 'things wrong':

> *"...em, my sister is there for me....she helps me to decide on things, yeah. I can't decide on my own. I don't want to get things wrong"*

Alison, statement also includes relying on her mum before she decides on things of importance, as she indicated that things could get 'confusing sometimes'

> *"I can't decide on my own, I have to call my mother. Things get confusing sometimes"*

Friends and colleagues also seemed to play a role in how participants made important decisions, as most participants also attributed the consultation with friends, including work colleagues as highly important in their decision making. For example, Gerald's statement included 'always' consulting with friends and colleagues before making important decisions, stating that one of the friends was 'always there' for him and reliance on his advice:

> *"But some of the people that I can say uhhh...ummm..that's important to me is the people that I work with and the*

people I help. I have got two good friends that I normally go and see and one of them is normally always there with me, giving me good advice..."

This existence of elements of reliance on others including family members and friends, referred to as significant others in decision making has been identified by literature (Cheng et al, 2013), as playing a role in the formation of externality in LOC. The participants' seemingly strong reliance on other members of the family before taking important decisions demonstrated in most of the responses seem to suggest that some level of externality exists in their perception of control over their lives, as they are not likely to take decisions on their own without consulting people outside of themselves. This also indicates that the majority of the participants' attitudes to taking decisions are in line with the character of collectivism (Cheng et al, 2013).

The foregoing also suggests that some element of externality may exist in the perception of most of the participants, as they are not likely to take total control of their own decisions without consulting people outside of themselves, most importantly, family and friends. The responses by the A & C participants seem to support the findings of the literature that BME members tend to rely on family members and significant others in their decision making, and suggests that they are likely to be external in their LOC. It also suggests that they are not likely to take decisions on their own without the confirmation or agreement with their family members or friends whom they consider important in their lives, which is an indication of externality in LOC. It also indicates that LOC needs to be considered in the context of their ethnicity and cultures.

1.2. Taking Decisions in Relation to Mental Health - Differences in Consultation- Avoidance Family and Friends

One subordinate theme that emanated from the participants' statements was in response to decision making relating to mental health. Under this subtheme, most of the participants differed in their responses under decision making when it relates to whom they would consult whenever they must take decisions regarding their mental health and any challenges that occur in this context. It describes the persons they consider as important to them, and therefore influence their decision making about mental health issues. It was found that although most participants referred to consulting family members, friends and even work colleagues before they take important decisions, most of the participants indicated that they avoid discussing their mental health challenges with members of the family and friends.

An example of this viewpoint is contained in Bianca's statement, as she expressed that she would not 'discuss it', and trying to 'be as normal as possible':

> *"I consult with people but when we're talking about my mental health; I don't discuss it. I always find that er.... I always find that um, it's not ready to do anything yet...you know, not as far as where you are and basically you try and be as normal as possible".*

It was found that most of the participants also expressed that they would not consult family members and friends in this context, but only those family members and friends who have experience of mental health challenges. This was an exception to the earlier observed responses that they would consult with family members and friends to make important decisions.

The importance of consulting with people with such experiences of mental health challenges was expressed in the context of their ability to demonstrate empathy and understanding in comparison to the response of people without such experiences. One example of this view is contained in the statement by Alison who expressed the importance of identifying with people of similar experiences and that only those people would be able to empathise with her due to having had similar experiences. She also indicated that identifying with people with personal experience of mental health issues are even preferred to the health professional or even a counsellor:

"People who have experienced erm.....situations similar to myself because they can identify with what you're going through and empathise rather than just a professional there who just writes a prescription or even somebody who is counselling you, if they cannot provide you with comparative experiences that they have lived through themselves it's almost impossible for them to empathise with you. They can sympathise with you, but they can't empathise with you so for me it's important to be talking to somebody who has experienced similar to what I have". (Alison, 1-1).

The expression of this view around having someone 'who can identify with' experiences of others suggests that people in this community are more likely to rely on advice from people with experience of mental health challenges within their own communities before taking decisions rather than a health professional. Another example of this perception was contained in Gerald's statement; he highlighted that such family members and friends with previous experience of mental health challenges could offer good example of confidence, 'structured' life and 'better decisions' in life:

"Well they'd be more confident in themselves um...they would make....they'd be more structured. They'd make better decisions in their life I believe erm..not to say they would make the right decisions but even if things did not go as planned they'd be able to modify their plan and still eventually get to their destination".(Gerald, 1-1).

This suggests that although most participants would consult with family and friends on general issues, they are likely to consult with those they perceived have some element of confidence and can therefore boost their own confidence to take decisions. This almost suggests a desire to rely on people whom they can not only have things in common with but seen as role models for taking decisions in relation to mental health.

The expression regarding being 'as normal as possible' seems to suggest a desire not to act in ways that would seem abnormal to family and friends, which emanated from the decision to avoid discussing mental health challenges. It would also connote that the reason behind the decision not to discuss the challenges was accompanied by a feeling of being abnormal while facing mental health challenges and a desire to appear normal. This suggests further that stigma about mental health may be an issue that plays a role in advice seeking before taking decision regarding mental health challenges by A & C groups. It also suggests that the internality in LOC may be due to a perception that they would rather not seek help or support on mental health issues from trusted people who are their family members and friends if they did not have any experience of mental health challenges.

1.3. Spirituality in Taking Decisions- Consultation with Pastors and Reliance on Prayers

One other subtheme within decision making is found in the expression of spiritual beliefs by most participants in this study. They expressed that their decisions on important issues are taken in consultation with their belief in the spiritual, including their own personal action of praying, as well as consulting religious leaders. Such expressions include the practice of taking their time in consulting such powers before making important decisions. An example of this view was expressed in a statement by Jane, who referred to having faith, a belief in 'The Father's superiority over human beings as well as praying in relation to making decisions:

> *"Normally, how I take decisions about important things in my life....erm...because, I have a Faith. I believe in The Father, someone who is more superior to human beings and when I pray and when I look at decisions and things surrounding decisions that I'm making; I think about it a long time before making that decision to be wise so that I make the right decision or near to the right one"* (Jane, 1-1).

Although most of the participants did not indicate how they receive confirmation regarding their decisions by consulting higher beings, their expressed view suggests also that their decisions are likely to be influenced by their beliefs. In another example, George expressed that his decisions are preceded by praying and waiting 'for some time' in this vein:

> *"I pray and I wait on myself for some time so I can say "that is the decision that I've come to"*

This belief in spirituality was also expressed in consulting with the church leaders before making decisions, as expressed by Carla that she would first contact her church pastor:

> *"Aaah, ahh I would go to the Pastor of my church"*

The expression of beliefs was also accompanied by not only prayers but also acknowledgement of God, as well as the importance of being close to God by attending churches and reading books, which are in turn expressed as contributed that their spirituality and helped them to cope. An example of this view is found in Alison's statement regarding attending church weekly:

> *"Being spiritual...I mean I go to church every week, but I buy books, read, go to church, say my prayers. You're closer to God this way at times. The constant battle of noise and, it's so much different. It's so much different".* (Alison, 1-1).

Another expression of faith God as a factor and importance in decision making was indicated in the context of being able to speak with the higher Being. An example of this view is found in Bianca's statement in which she drew an analogy of medication and talking therapies, indicating that 'having a good relationship with God' and being able to 'offload':

> *"...faith helps as well, it's not just about medication or talking therapies. It's also about having a good relationship with God so that you can offload on somebody. You don't have to*

> *psychically have to have somebody there in person to speak to, you can speak to God".* (Bianca, 1-1)

The belief in the spiritual and its role in decision making was also expressed by Alan who expressed having no power over his own life, a failure over decisions, and importance of faith as follows:

> *"Well I've got no power over my own life that's first and foremost, because I make decisions and make plans but sometimes it doesn't work out. Um...so..that's not me doing it, it's coming from a different source and because of my faith again, I believe it's coming from a higher source than mankind. I say it's my Father, that's why I call it my Father, in my faith I call him the unseen spirit and ....gives me..."*

It was also found that the participants combine both consulting with others along with resorting to prayers before making decisions. One example of this view was expressed by Brian as follows:

> *"I seek advice, I pray".*

This suggests that many participants believe in supernatural forces and would choose to rely on those forces in their decision making. This also connotes some externality in LOC, as it suggests that their decision making is influenced by powers outside of themselves which they believe can have an impact on their fate. The acknowledgement of the existence of God, reliance on prayers and developing a relationship with God expressed by the participants in relation to decision making raises issue around spirituality and the experience of mental health clients in the A & C populations with services. One of these issues relates to the extent to which the spirituality of clients is considered by health professionals, and if such expression of spiritual beliefs has negative or positive relationship to the decision-making process and consequently the welfare of the clients in the care settings.

1.4. Summary –Theme 1

The foregoing subordinate topics which emanated from the perception of control around decision making have demonstrated that most participants took into consideration several factors before making decisions on important issues. It was found that most participants expressed that the factors depend on the type of the decisions to be made. Two categories of decisions have arisen from the responses in this study- decisions about general issues of importance and decisions about mental health challenges. They would rely on family members and friends and consult them before making decisions regarding issues that are not connected to mental health challenges. On the other hand, their reliance on other people including family and friends for advice does not extend to mental health issues. Their decision to avoid discussing mental health challenges with friends and family members was due to their perception that those friends and friends would not understand the challenges except where they have experience of similar challenges. It would also suggest that stigma may play a role in this regard, as there seem to be attempts to appear 'normal'. Consequently, the participants would only discuss their mental health issues with people with experience of mental health challenges. Participants would also consult their religious leaders such as pastors while others believe in a higher being and resort to prayers. This expression of belief and consultation with religious leaders seem to suggest that the participants perceive that certain issues in their lives were beyond their control and they required advice regarding decision making about such issues. Making decisions by consulting others first including family members, friends, religious leaders and prayers also indicate some elements of externality in LOC. One could also conclude that most participants expressed some internality in LOC when it comes to mental health issues, as they avoid consulting other people, except those they believe have similar experiences; in which case their external LOC in this regard is limited, as it is based on their taking control by indicating the criteria of the people they would consult for advice before making decisions. This means that in making decisions, there is a combination of expressed internality and externality in LOC by the participants - higher externality for general issues other than mental health, and a higher level of internality with regards to mental health issues. It could also be read that the participants were not feeling powerless in relation to mental health, which may not be considered a negative thing to have a perception of control. However, such perceived control may also result in negative outcome by not seeking help and support from family members and friends on time, until crisis points and coercive entry pathways to mental health services. The findings here also raise the issues around spirituality playing a role in the decisions service users from these A & C populations make regarding their lives and mental health.

2| Perception of Levels of Control in Relation to Mental Illness Experience

This superordinate theme contains subtopics that encompass the participants' perception of control of their lives. The perception of control was elicited by asking the participants their views around control over their lives, what being in control of one's life meant to them, and the extent to which they felt that they were in control over their lives. The findings indicate that the participants expressed their perception of whether they have control of their lives in relation to their experience of mental health challenges. Their perceptions in this regard were expressed in terms of level of control as opposed to expressing what control means and decision making as indicated in the first superordinate theme.

The subtopics under this include the level of control they perceived as relating to mental illness triggers, those experienced during mental hospital admission process, their experience of hospital stay and discharge, and experience after discharge. It contains subtopics that emanated from the responses, including their view of loss of control over their lives, which most of the participants attributed to being contributory or acting as triggers to their mental illness experience; perceived loss of identity as having been attributed to their mental illness experiences; differences in view of control over their lives between admission process and hospitalisation, their hospital and discharge experiences, and post hospital discharge experience; all of which elicited varying levels of perception of control.

2. 1. Level of Control – Stress Factors as Mental Illness Triggers

Under this sub theme, most participants expressed their view on the meaning of having control over one's life by narrating their experiences prior to what they described as a mental breakdown. They likened being in control over their lives to the conditions of their lives prior to the commencement of the experiences that they expressed caused stresses to their daily living. They attributed a loss of control of their lives to the stresses that they identified as challenges to their mental health which led to hospitalisation. Some participants also attributed this perceived lack of control of their lives due to the stressors and conditions as factors which led to their mental illness experiences.

One aspect of this lack of control was expressed in relation to the experience of stress at work and challenges with coping with work demands. Alison described a strain of work demands including long hours of work:

> *"From work.... It was a strain. I used to do a lot of hours, used to start at 7 in the morning and finish at 9 at night and it's catering and it's constant.....all the time".* (Alison, 1-1)

Carla also described the experience of breakdown due to long hours of work, also expressing a surprise that she survived:

> *".....it leads to the breakdown... umm....I was doing a lot of hours and I wasn't eating well and um...it was a constant thing of worrying all day and you don't realise the pressure. I'm still shocked that I'm still here".* (Carla, FG2)

These suggest that the stresses of work demands and their impact on the feeling of control or a feeling of not being able to cope with the demands of work may constitute an externality in LOC, as the participants could have experienced lacking control over their lives as a result of those stresses. As these pressures and demands of the daily routines contributed to mental health challenges for most of the participants, it would also suggest that a feeling of not being able to cope could have been considered a sign of failure leading further to externality in their LOC.

Another aspect of the stressors that were expressed by most of the participants as having led to them feeling a lack of control over their lives, and which led to mental health problems was the expressed pressure from their superiors in addition to work demands. For example, Patricia described having one's 'structure' being used all day, and the action of a 'boss':

> *"It was a pressure because sometimes you had to be on your own and work on your own and there was a lot of ummm....deliveries and stuff like that to do and you know your whole structure is being used all day.......... well.... someone tends to be more of a boss than you are..you know, stepping all over you, inconsiderate".* (Patricia, FG1)

Some of the participants also perceived that a feeling of having their lives being taken over by someone else, rather than their own actions (external LOC), as having contributed to their mental illness experience. An example of this perception is contained in Alison's description of her experience at work in which she expressed feeling that someone else had taken over her life:

> *"I couldn't say the lead to this was my own actions, I couldn't say that. Like if it's my own actions it means that someone took over and I wasn't around. Simple"* (1-1).

Having a feeling of someone else taking over one's life is also an expression of externality in LOC, as it indicates from Alison's statement also that she perceived that she 'wasn't around'.

Some participants also expressed losing control over their lives due to perception that their lives were being controlled by others. Brian explained that he felt that addictions, including alcohol and drugs played a part in his view of not being in control:

> *"In the past it's been all external, a lot of external things have controlled me....erm...well I didn't have control over my life because of my addictions. My life was unmanageable basically and my mental health...it was unmanageable...(due to) ...alcohol and drugs"* (FG1)

The expression of the perception of loss of control was also explained by many of the participants as being due to a combination of factors including pressure in the work place due to feeling exhaustion, frustration, discrimination and a perceived lack of promotion, and perceived poor prospects in career advancement. One example of these factors is contained in the statement by Patricia who described a feeling of 'being suppressed', a feeling of low prospect for career progression in spite of being told that she possessed necessary skills and ability, not being given managerial roles, which she further described led to 'burnout':

> *".....the fact that I was being suppressed in the work place and erm....I was always told that I had the skills and ability but promotion was erm....what they call that glass ceiling and it just wasn't happening. I would be erm...you know...in the presence of absence or in the.... you know...anything like that; I would be called upon to carry out the role but actually having the role in a full time capacity wasn't going to happen. It became disheartening and it leads to....it leads to burnout really... that's the...that's the correct diagnosis for it. It was burnout".*

This experience was also expressed in relation to the consequences of those factors which were considered frustrating by Patricia, which then led to depression, inability to control mood, thoughts and judgement, which in turn led to mental illness experience:

> *"Burnout leads to severe depression.... severe depression leads to inability to control one's thoughts, one's mood, one's overall judgement; everything just kind of......... Because it's a ...it's a grinding down. It doesn't happen overnight it's a continuous grinding down of the person's strength until the person is unable to function and then.... you end up severely ill"* (FG1).

These suggest that the feelings of these factors were indicative of a lack of control and externality in LOC, which led to mental illness experience for, many of the participants who were working before they became mentally ill.

The expression of the attribution of racial discrimination as precursor to and contributory to their mental illness experience was also a constant feature in most of the participants' description of what it meant to lack control over one's life. An example of this position is indicated in Mary's statement in which she described experience of 'racism and prejudice', being 'over the edge' which resulted in 'breakdown' and having to stay with a friend from which she had to also see a psychiatrist:

> *"But the major thing that really, really sent me over the edge...remember racism and prejudice based on culture and belief ......just doesn't start at one particular point. It starts from the year dot, it's continuous; and it breaks you down and it breaks you up inside and it mashes up your head.....he phoned my friend and she came and got me in the pub and I stayed in bed for about 2 weeks in her house and that was the real start of what I call my breakdown. That was it from there and from there I had to go and see a psychiatrist, the doctor came and take me to the psychiatrist..."* (1-1)

The experience of racism was also expressed as being contributory to a lack of career advancement. For example, Carla expressed being denied opportunity because of the colour of her skin, and that advancement in her career would have been achieved if she had not been discriminated against in the workplace:

> *"Well, I actually feel that if I had had been a white British...I would have made it because ...I know and I know that because I was there. So, I erm..I feel that based....I was denied an opportunity based on my skin colour".* (FG2)

The experience of racism was also expressed in the parlance of leading to frustration and unemployment as a result of not being able to cope and having to take the decision to leave employment. An example of this lack of control due to perceived discrimination on account of race was in the statement expressed by Alan who described leaving his employment due to racism:

> *"Well my reaction was gradually erm... frustration and annoyance and stress and erm...gradually.....leaving the post".* (1-1)

The loss of employment due to racism could have in turn led to further loss of control of one's life's finances, which could in turn have led to their breakdown. These are also indicative of externality in LOC.

The experience of racism as being a contributory factor in expression of a lack of control was also discussed by many participants from the context of their childhood experiences. Many expressed that the experience of racial abuse during their childhood years led to a feeling of a lack of confidence and self-esteem as well as a feeling that they had no control over their lives. Most of the participants also expressed that they attributed their mental illness experiences to have been caused by the racial abuse from their childhood years. An example of this view is contained in Alison's statement in which she described experiencing racism, and suffering from anxiety when young:

> *"... I had a lot of racist, I had a lot of racial problems and erm.....I had a lot of anxiety. I suffered from anxiety from a young age".* (1-1)

Brian also expressed having to report to his family his experience of racial abuse when he was growing up:

> *"Well how I was brought up, the way I was brought up; because I had so much abuse...racial abuse....I would come in crying to my family saying "someone called me a blackie or a nigger" or something like that. I used to have terrible things said to me"* (Brian, FG1).

The experience of racism and bullying during younger years was also expressed as having impacted on the feeling of a loss of control over one's life by many of the participants. This was also expressed as a factor that led to mental health challenges in later years, even as most of the participants also described having experienced some form of mental health challenges from a young age. An example of this view was Carla and her experience of bullying and racism which led to anxiety, resulting in being placed on medication at a 'young age'. She also expressed a feeling of being treated as just a 'young black girl', a lack of empathy and not being offered counselling:

> *"From that young age I was on medications and the way I was treated was like "oh she's just a young black girl" and this and that "she'll be alright". There was no counselling, there was no empathy, there was no understanding of who I was or what was going on for me; anything like that and the reason why I was anxious. The reason why I was anxious was because I was being bullied and being taunted and you know racial things and stuff like that. Their answer was to give me medication and that would take away the anxiety".* (FG2)

A similar experience was expressed by another participant, as being contributory to their mental illness experience. This was also illustrated in the context of how the causative experience has extended to their feeling a loss of control and a sense of dependency after discharge from hospital:

> *"Well essentially my mental illness has been caused by predominantly traumatic events in my life. Bullying at school, mistreatment by mother's neighbours and stuff like that ..."* (Dwayne, 1-1)

These expressions and the accompanied sample statements indicate that the participants were predominantly undergoing a high level of loss of control over their lives as a result of the various stressors outlined. It suggests also that their LOC were on the high externality scale, which led to their mental illness experiences as well as contact with the services. The expressions of experiencing 'frustration and annoyance and stress', 'bullying at school', 'being taunted' and references to 'traumatic events' are likely factors that could lead to a perception of a loss of control in one's life. It thus suggests that many of the participants were placed in the externality end of the internal-external LOC spectrum before their contact with the services. It also indicates that some of them were also fallen within the externality spectrum from a young age as a result of the experience of racism.

2.2. Level of Control – Perceived Challenges Regarding Identity as Factor in Mental Illness Experience

In addition to the expressed view of a lack of control over their lives as a result of stresses explained earlier, most of the participants also expressed the role played by a perceived lack of identity. The perceived loss of identity was adduced as a factor that did not only contribute to their mental illness experiences but became an integral part of their mental health challenges. Loss of identity was, therefore, illustrated as being responsible in part for their perceived loss of control over their lives. In this respect, many of the participants explained that having been born and growing up in Great Britain, and failing to find creative avenues and "services" that would enable them to explore their interests as men and women of A & C backgrounds also led to confusion regarding where they belonged, frustration, anger and a feeling of a lack of cultural identity. An example of this perception is included in Mary's statement, which included a feeling that she was also controlled:

> *"Well I was a very confused person, I had no identity; I didn't know my identity and I was controlled. My people and the authorities controlled me, I had no say, I had no say".* (1-1).

This also suggests experience of a challenge with having a sense of belonging, as it has also been posited that identity, which describes how one knows oneself and how one is known to others as well as identifying with groups, are important to mental health (Haslam et al, 2009). This challenge was also described by Brian who expressed making effort to find his own identity, but which was hampered by his struggle with his mental health challenges:

> *"I felt it was very important for me to formulate my identity but at the time I was half in half out in terms of my own mind because I was struggling with mental illness at the same time and I didn't know it you know".* (1-1).

Another example of this view of loss of control due to identity loss, which, in turn, led to mental illness and hospitalisation, is contained in an excerpt from Ryan's (1-1) interview. He described a perceived loss of identity and isolation, due to a lack of what he referred to as 'services' as playing a role in his mental illness experience:

> *".... contributed to me having a mental health issue...my experience was umm....ummm... I lost control. I lost control of my identity. I had my identity in the days when I was growing up but somewhere along the way when I grew up. I started to mix a bit more at my own pace in the community. I did get isolated at one time because services at that time weren't around. The services that I wanted to obtain weren't around. I had to make do with whatever was available which wasn't what I was looking for so....erm...I was looking for something a little more creative, something a little more outstanding, something that could help people.."* (1-1)

Alan also described his struggles with finding facilities that could enable him to explore his interests and find his identity, and the view that he did not receive the support he wanted. In citing the example of the level of education he had attained to affirm to himself that he was not 'stupid' he also expressed that he felt that he was treated 'like a child' instead of being provided the support he was looking for:

> *"It's very difficult you know, you know I have got two degrees in my time, One in law and the other in biomedical science, which I didn't complete for various reasons, because I became ill or gave up for various reasons. So, what I'm trying to say is I'm not stupid. So, it's really difficult to find facilities who really cater for me you know, in terms of my identity, my interests, you know they were trying to be nice to me but I remember they were talking to me like a child you know? I was 38 years of age. People are affected differently, and people react differently you know"* (1-1).

The loss of identity was also linked with the role culture played in the perceived loss of control that was expressed by most of the participants. In expressing their hospital experiences, most of the participants also linked their view of a lack of control from the context that their culture which was part of their identity was not acknowledged. For example, Adrian described the impact of his hospital experience in relation to having nothing to remind him of his culture. He also explained the importance of culture as the 'root' of himself, how he becomes different without it, describing that as 'someone else', 'a different me', as well as its importance to his identity. He also expressed a desire to gain his identity again, and recognise his heritage and tradition:

> *"Whilst I was locked up in the hospital on the ward there was nothing there and no one there to remind me of my culture. As I said, the root of myself is my culture and if the root is not there, it's not me, it's someone else; it's a different me. So the root has to come back for me to grow again and to gain my identity again and to recognise my heritage and tradition"*. (FG1)

The foregoing indicates that most of the participants perceived that their LOC were highly external due to the influence of their perception of a loss of control. This perception was also expressed as being due to their view of a loss of identity, the lack of control over their identity, as well as a lack of support to enable them to explore their identity. This includes a perceived lack of creative avenues as well as services through which they could be able to explore and regain the identity they perceived to have been lost. This perception also seemed to be exacerbated by their mental health challenges. They also expressed their hospital experiences in which they reported that they were unable to find things and people to which they could relate with culture; this seems to also contribute to their feeling of a loss of their identity as their culture was integral to their sense of identity. These expressions confirm the literature position that a feeling of that one is not able to exert an influence on issues in one's life is an indication for externality in LOC.

2.3. Differences in Perceptions of Control - Pre and Post Hospital Admission and Discharge

Within this subtheme many participants related their perception of control to their experiences with services during their mental health journeys. It contains their views regarding control over their lives from two different contexts- hospital admission and stay and their post discharge experience. It comprises the expression of the sense of control they perceived during their hospital admissions, including the process that led to their hospitalisation for treatment, their hospital stays on the one hand, and their perception of LOC following their discharge from hospital on the other. The various stages of experiences were expressed by most participants as being different from each other, which, in turn, placed their perceptions on different levels of LOC.

2.3.1. Admission Process and Hospital Experience

Most of the participants' description of their hospital experiences were characterised by a feeling of a lack of control. This includes the admission process in which many of them expressed that their opinions were not considered. An example of this view is included in Dwayne's narration of his first experience of admission which involved the police. He described having no control but experience of having his door 'kicked down', being accused of doing things and then being given injection against his will:

> *"The first time they put me in hospital they took me in there in my underwear... they wouldn't even let me put my clothes on when they came. They just kicked the door down and just rushed in and they just started talking all this rubbish about all these things I didn't do...... Then I was in the shower with the door kicked off and I said to them "well if you're going to take me away, I expect you to let me put my clothes on and you can take me away. They took me out of the place in my underwear, put me in the unit, took off my underwear, gave me an injection, I fell asleep and woke up on the ward...."* (1-1).

The view of a lack of control (external LOC) indicated in not being able to have their view expressed, heard or taken into consideration also appear to be further exacerbated by the hospital stay experiences, as the participants' sense of lack of control were described from the ambit of having no say or any control over decisions. Alan's statement includes an example of this view, in which he narrated being taken away when his mother called a doctor to 'examine' him, which was then followed by police being called, and things happening 'so fast'. He also indicated that he was 'still trying to have a say':

> *"On my admission to the mental health hospital, which was some years ago now I had no control over it, I had no say in it at all. A short excerpt from my story is that I was at my mum's place having dinner and she called the doctor in to examine me, the police came, and they took me in the ambulance to*

the mental health hospital. I didn't have a say in it all, everything happened so fast and the mechanism that was in place was that I didn't have a say in it and to this day I'm still trying to have a say in it even though it all happened a long time ago. So what I'm doing now to help with this PhD and this interview um...is of benefit to me as well umm... to speak up about what happened to me you know erm... and for someone to say well this is awful, or this is good or this is something you know? Erm.... I had no control". (1-1).

This narrated experience which included an expression of a desire for someone to comment on their experience seems to be a need for a validation, and also seems to indicate that the participants still feel that their voices are not being heard even after a lapse in time since their admission into hospital.

These views expressed by the participants regarding not being in control during the admission process seem to be exacerbated during their period of stay in hospital. Most participants expressed a perception of continued loss of control whilst in hospital, including a lack of involvement in decisions about their treatment. An example of this view is contained in Dwayne's statement in which he describes his experience regarding decisions being made on his behalf without being asked. He also indicated externality in LOC in his response to that experience, his way of stating his opinion without challenging decisions made for him in order to manage his situation, as felt that his perceived condition of a lack of influence on the decisions would not have changed if they had been challenged by him:

"...decisions were made for me and the only way I could influence them is by....is by...well, basically agreeing to what had been said and then coming back and saying my opinion on what that decision was. So, I did learn to....I didn't really challenge any decisions because that wouldn't have helped the situation I don't feel. I was better off trying it, coming

back and saying why I agreed with it or disagreed with it".(1-1).

Another participant also expressed that the lack of say into the decision made by the health care professionals for them to be put on some medication regime made them feel that they had lost control of their lives. An example of this view was expressed by Dennis' statement in which he described having 'no say', being forced to take medication, and feeling like a baby:

> *"I had no say in the medication they forced me to take. I was like a baby because of the medication which I called a spiritual strait jacket."* (FG1)

This expression of externality in LOC in feeling of having a 'spiritual strait jacket' seems like an indication of being restrained in a spiritual sense, which could also be interpreted as feeling a loss of control both physically and spiritually. Noella used a similar expression of having 'no control' of her life in hospital, she also indicated that she found that she had to do what resulted from the situation where 'decisions were made' for her. She also expressed that she felt that 'power came in' for her when she decided that she had to leave the hospital:

> *".. I had no control of my life when I was in hospital and decisions were made for me and I had to do that but power came in for me when I made the decision that I'm not staying in hospital. "I don't know what's going to happen, what's going to take place, I don't want to stay in hospital, I want to go home" I tried as good as I could and see the outcome..."* (1-1).

The expression regarding power also seems to suggest that the participant might have felt 'powerless' from the experience of having decisions made on her behalf without her control, to the extent that she felt that she had to draw on 'power' (internality in LOC), by summoning courage to take the decision to leave the hospital, although she did not 'know what was going to happen'.

Another example of the view of externality in LOC due to a perception of lack of control is contained in Alison's statement in which she also described the impact of the experience of hospitalisation has had on her. She expressed finding it difficult to speak about it even after discharge, being stirred up, being unable to 'get over it', and having to 'walk around the streets just to make sure':

> *"It sits on you and stirs you up um... it's just hard talking about it because you're not that far from it...it's not like it happened, it took place and you get over it. You can't really get over it because there are so many things going on, so many things attached to it. From home to hospital it's different, just to...just to.... I have to walk around the streets just to make sure, just to know... I'm around my place....I'm by myself that I'm not with people like I used to and I find I get tired but you know it needs to be...it needs to be with people that can explain"* (1-1).

These expressions also seem to indicate that the level of externality in LOC had been so high to the extent that the participant felt that they had to be reassured that they were 'free' after being discharged. It also gives further indication to the effect that most of the participants described a difference in their perception of a lack of control between their experiences whilst on hospital admission in comparison to their experience when they were discharged.

2.3.2. Post Hospital Experience – Contradictory and Different Levels of Control of Life's Situation

In this subtheme, most of the many participants described a feeling of gaining control over their lives after getting discharged from hospitals. This sense of control was in the parlance of being able to make decisions. One example of this is contained in Jane's statement in which she also expressed that she could no longer be controlled, dictated to, as well as finding herself and her own identity:

> *"Well obviously I feel that I've found myself now and my identity and I feel that I'm able to speak up a bit more for myself now and things like that and they can't dictate to me....they can't control me. They used to be able to do that in the past"* (Jane, FG1).

These expressions seem to indicate that the perception of a loss of control within the hospital experience is also being linked to a perceived loss of self and loss of identity as an African or Caribbean individual. This link also seems to be in line with the expression of loss of identity or challenges regarding identity as being a trigger to the illness experience described under the perception of control topics.

Another expression of sense of control after discharge from hospital is also found in Carla's statement in which she described being 'pretty in control':

> *"Oh yeah, I feel as I'm pretty in control yeah, yeah....Erm....with my mental health, with my physical health to a degree. I mean there are certain things that will come up with my physical health that it's just natural and wear and tear as they say. My housing situation is under control, my financial situation is under control. My day to day living is under control"* (Carla, FG2).

This also indicates that a feeling of control of one's life is linked to having situations such as housing and finance 'under control', thereby further suggesting that a perceived control over these issues are indicators of LOC internality from these participants' perspectives.

However, majority of the participants also expressed that they later found that the perceived sense of control was short-lived, as they found themselves to be highly dependent on others for daily living activities and for their livelihood:

> *"To a degree I'm in control and in part I'm not in control because like I said it's this medication. If I come off this*

medication, I'm scared. I don't know what would happen to me so I feel that I am controlled by the system to stay on the medication and to another extent I could try to come off the medication slowly with the help of the professional people.....and see what happens". (Carla, FG2)

Another participant also mentioned feeling a loss of control due to dependency on medication:

> *"To a degree that I am and to a degree I feel that I'm not because I'm on medication now permanently and I feel like I'm not in control and not in charge because I feel that the medication is in charge of me".* (Tim, FG2).

One of the participants described a lack of control post discharge from hospital from a feeling of a sense of boredom and an inability to make sense of the world, and having to depend on other people:

> *"...but I .... with the boredom that's actually built up over my life over the years um....you still need someone talking to you, you still need someone that's normal ummm....making sense for you. You still need all that, you don't know what's sensible really, you don't know what's sensible".* (Dwayne, 1-1).

In further response to the question regarding what it means to be in control of one's life, majority of the participants indicated that it was necessary to be able to cope with daily activities both physically and emotionally, be confident and financially independent. An example of this view of control over life is included in Tim's statement in which he described several factors to be accomplished, including financial, maintenance of physical and mental health, assertiveness and confidence in their relationship with health professionals:

> *"To be in control of one's life, we can live from day to day ...maintain our house if we've got one, maintain our life,*

> *maintain bills erm. .maintain mental and physical health. Be able to socialise, be able to interact, be able to stand up for oneself when we need to, be assertive, be confident and let the doctors and the mental health team....to be able to make them aware of who we are and our capabilities and needs and things like that and that we are in control".*(FG2).

This seems to indicate that participants considered that some specific factors are prerequisite to being 'in control'. It also suggests that internality in LOC is linked with the ability of people to be able to achieve self-management including maintain a combination of financial, physical, mental, self-confidence, and social interactions. These, however, seem to be lacking in the description of most participants' experiences which included a feeling of powerlessness after discharge. An example of this experience is included in Dylan's statement in which he expressed that the long period of admission had led to him becoming confused and unable to decide on how to control his life's situation when he was discharged. He described a lack of people to socialise with, 'having no control', and a feeling of helplessness that what he expected to get support from the doctors did not 'seem to work':

> *"After such a long time in that place, having no control I felt....um.... I was mad. I wasn't able to think about getting back. I've been brought this way and what am I going to do, what am I going to do? I don't know anyone, I just don't know. I expected to be in more with doctors and stuff like that but um...it doesn't seem to work that way"* (1-1).

In addition, many of the participants also expressed feeling of a loss of control in relation to finances and being dependent on the government for survival. For example, Melanie expressed an inability to gain control of her finances as well as regain her career due to the long time spent in hospital; she also described the impact of the medication resulting in making her feel like a 'zombie':

> *".... I mean, I was not in control, couldn't get any more career, and the psychiatrist, as I have said, those bloody tablets she gave me half killed me anyway. And, I ended up like a bloody zombie on benefits".* (FG2).

These expressions indicate a high level of externality in LOC, including a feeling of helplessness, a loss of confidence due to long period of hospitalisation, a feeling of a poor prospect in regaining one's career, and a feeling of dependency.

The link between the post discharge experiences and the perceived lack of control was also expressed by most of the participants from the perspective of the need for the stresses that contributed to the mental illness experiences to be addressed to enable them to regain control over their lives. Furthermore, most of the participants expressed an inability to secure and retain gainful employment due to their mental illness experience and the associated ongoing stresses which impacted on their ability to secure gainful employment and maintain their mental health. For example, Alison's statement below described a scenario in which someone has received good mental health support but the benefit of which is hampered by what she described as 'those stresses still in the community':

> *"...so again going to a psychiatric hospital yes you're mended you're well, you're given all the support and the psychological help and you're on the right balance of medication but if those stresses are still in the community, unless you have developed coping mechanisms or a way to accept that or deal with it you're always going to be fighting against it and end up ill or you are just going to become subdued and accept what's happened so it doesn't seem like a win, win situation".* (1-1).

This suggests that the impact of the challenges experienced in relation to social issues of unemployment and other social inequalities (Williams & Keating, 2005), are likely to impact on people's LOC in both general and mental health contexts, even if they had received satisfactory medical support. It also suggests an association of these issues with stigma and discrimination relating to mental illness which also gives the clients the feeling of what has been described as an absence of a *'win, win situation'*. Another example of this view is included in Brian's statement in which he expressed that there was a low likelihood that clients who are recovering would be able to meet the expectations of achieving employment, as they also have to focus on getting well whilst exploring their employment prospects.

> *"Because you know just as any healthy person, you know mentally stable person can be all sorts of different people they seem to be putting all the mental health sort of down route to this kind of average and it's not going to be...I mean most people are just not going to be shop cashiers or whatever when they're, when they're well. They're going to be creative people or constructive people or social and there doesn't seem to be any option other than get well".* (FG1).

This also indicates that clients focus on regaining their mental health as a priority while they also have interest in regaining some gainful employment. However, the latter is hampered by the illness experience. The LOC in this regard also seems to be external, as the clients seem to be grappling with both trying to remain mentally stable while going through the expectation that he/she also needs to get into employment. This is further expressed in most of the participants' description of feeling vulnerable to expectations that they seek employment, as it is a condition for receiving social support that they demonstrate that they are actively seeking employment. This condition has also been expressed as exerting pressure on them in their recovery journeys. An example of this view is contained in Carla statement in which she described a sense of frustration at being asked to 'go to the job centre' while she was only becoming stable and having a bit of 'control':

> *"That's it. Just get well and once you're a little bit well, once you have a little bit of control it's like "ok, go to the job*

> *centre, there are the jobs there so go and mess up your life..." and then you're back to square one".* (FG2).

This position also suggests that the clients are likely to feel a state of externality in LOC as a result of the expectation that they should be seen to be actively looking for employment after discharge, even when they did not feel that they were in enough control to handle the situation of seeking employment or even being able to secure or retain it. It also suggests that the working of the benefit system may have some negative impact on the post-hospital experiences, as the participants have also articulated that cuts in social welfare negatively affect their recovery.

This perception of externality is also further expressed from the point of view that the clients' sense of externality in LOC is indicated in a sense of dependency on the state and the conditions that must be met to receive benefits to survive financially. An example of this view is highlighted by Trish, who described the procedure and conditions that accompany receiving State support, and describing the fear of ending up 'in trouble' as a result of failure to comply with the conditions:

> *"You have to claim benefits and in order to claim benefits ...and in order to claim benefits you have to comply with job centre, you have to comply with your GP, you have to go to the GP and the psychiatrist to get the letters to support your claim...you have to do everything otherwise you just end up in trouble".* (FG2).

This seems to suggest that there is the existence of underlying fear of failure to comply with conditions of receiving benefits, which could lead to being denied financial support and consequently not being in control over their finances. The externality in LOC is also suggested here due to the expressed risk of benefits sanctions, as opposed to the view of internality that accompany discharge from hospital.

Most of the participants also expressed feeling dependent on the State due to unemployment, which they also see as intruding into their ability to control their lives. An example of this is included in Dwayne's statement in which he described that his mental illness experience has led to him having no other choice than to be dependent on state welfare. He also described this condition as constituting 'interference' in his life:

> *"Well I am dependant on the government for my finance, for my benefits and I'm dependant on the government for my medication which I need. So, society plays a big interference in my life…".* (1-1).

Another example of this view of dependency due to reliance on state benefits is indicated in Ryan's statement in which he describes LOC from the parlance of 'limitation to the control' he has on his life:

> *"On the other side of things, there is a limitation to the control that I have because, you know, been on Benefits to take somebody else's money. Somebody else kind a make that decision as how much you can get. So, you don't have kind a have control because of my mental illness. You have kind a limited by the way that I can live my life. So, that put a limitation. So, you can't live the way you, that you intend to your full potential. Also, I am living in rented accommodation, supported housing. I am kind a living in somebody else's property. So, you are living by somebody else's standards and not your own. You are not living in an environment that you would ideally choose to live. So, there is always that kind of limitation. At the same time, it is kind of sits within me to break free of all that. Kind of live life more in a way that I want to where you know, living to my full potential, doing my own thing".* (1-1).

This narrative describes factors of externality of LOC from mental health context, including other people making decision on one's behalf, and sometimes having to 'live in somebody else's standards', having no control as a result of mental illness experience, and a feeling that one is not living in an accommodation setting of their choice. The desire to 'break free' to 'live to own potential' and do one's own thing, as expressed here also indicates a realisation of the externality in LOC in the mental health context whilst recognising the challenges in this regard.

Patrick also described a feeling of partial level of control over his life. This was expressed in the context that the sense of incomplete control was due to not having his own home, as he is in supported housing and receiving benefits, which he described as being at the mercy of other entities:

> *"...but I also think that not feeling any control kind of keeps it perpetuating further because yes in a lot of ways I do feel ummm kind of control or are or kind of at the mercy of others. I mean because kind of you know I mean I live in. I'm on benefits, I'm on supported housing and so you're kind of living on somebody else's money and somebody else's property. It's like you know...that in order to live..."* (FG1).

These further suggest that there is some element of externality in LOC expressed by most of the participants, as they felt that they were unable to exert the type of control they would have wanted over their lives due to the influence of others. The externality also seems to be ongoing in their post hospital experiences of mental health.

2.4. Summary-Theme 2

The foregoing subtopics have described the perception of control of the participants from their mental health experiences, including their hospital and their post discharge contexts. The experiences seem to indicate perception of control in two seemingly contradictory contexts. On the one hand, most of the participants seem to indicate that they had gained a sense of control after getting discharged from hospital, which they expressed, were mostly not available to them in their experience whilst in hospital. Most expressions of externality in LOC have also been demonstrated by most of the participants in the foregoing superordinate and subtopics that relate to triggers of their mental illness experiences as well as the levels of control they experienced in the admission process, their hospitalisation and the period following their discharge. This includes the expression that their views were not taken into consideration in decisions taken by the health professionals and a feeling of incarceration. Other issues which were included in other topics include expression of a lack of inclusion of their family and friends' views and inputs in their treatment regime, the lack of attention to their culture in decision made about their health. These issues pointed to externality in their LOC from which they expressed that they had regained their control over when they were discharged. Their experience of discharge from hospital was, therefore, perceived as a state of regaining control over their lives in their mental health (internal LOC), as they expressed that they felt that they were able to take decisions regarding their lives that were not possible whilst on admission. The expression of a sense of control (internality in LOC), after getting discharged from hospital seems to have been based on a feeling of being free from restrictions with regards to movement as well as a feeling that they were able to exert some level of control on certain decisions regarding their daily living activities. They also expressed feeling in control on discharge, as they were also able to take care of themselves without having to wait on other people for some daily living activities. This also seems to be an expression of internality after getting discharged from hospital.

However, their post hospital experiences are also expressed in the context of some misgivings with regards to the view that their perception of control was not complete. In this context, they seem to have expressed a sense of contradiction between internality and externality in their LOC. The externality was expressed from the point of view that although they were physically free from the rules and regulations of hospital experiences, they viewed their perceived freedom to be limited by several factors. These include feeling of dependence on the state for their benefits, a feeling that they have low employment prospects as a result of their mental illness experiences, the stigma that accompanied the challenges relating to inability to attain gainful employment, the impact of medication on their health, as well as their ability to hold down employment and meet the demand of gainful employment. Other issues that seem to connote externality in the LOC of the participants include the perception that they were not in control of their benefits, as they had to abide by certain rules and regulations in order to receive benefits rather than being able to support themselves financially via gainful employment. They have also expressed feeling a lack of control due to the fear of readmission as a result of relapse, which, in turn, plays a role in their perception that they were dependent on medication, without which they feared that they might not get well or remain stable. All these factors point to externality in LOC. It, thus, suggests that the perception of a combination of internality and externality is demonstrated in the post hospital experiences of most of the participants in this study.

3| The Role of Culture in LOC

This superordinate theme contains the indications of the views expressed by the study participants in response to the question regarding the extent to which they felt that culture played a role in their perception of control over their lives. Most of the participants expressed that there was a relationship between their perception of control and their culture. This relationship was also expressed in relation to their treatment experience within mental health services, in which it is predominantly perceived that their culture was not considered in treatment experiences. This they, in turn, see as being the reason for their feeling that they had no control over their situation. The subtopics under this perception includes the significance of culture on identity, the importance of family and community, and the study participants' expressed view that the mental health services have a low perception of the cultures of A& C groups. These were also perceived to be responsible for their sense of inequality in their mental health experiences on account of culture, and externality in their LOC.

3.1. Significance of Culture in Identity and LOC

This subtheme contains the link made by participants between their culture and their perception of identity, which they consider as important factors in their perception of control over their lives. In response to the prompt question as to whether they perceived there was a link between their culture and their perception of identity, most of the participants commented on the importance of culture in relation to their identity as service users from A & C populations, by highlighting a link between the two concepts by expressing that their culture was an integral part of their identity. An example of this view is indicated by Dwayne, in which he described differences in use of language for different situations and audiences:

> *"...sometimes we talk in a different way to someone else and with people I know in the patois part of my community I talk with in a certain dialect. This is different from when I speak with other people"* (1-1).

This example of expressing oneself in dialect and patois (a Caribbean mode of expression) with people of similar culture in a different way from people from different parts highlights the role a difference in culture plays, and the importance of this to the participants' concept of identity. An example of this view was also indicated in Dwayne's statement in which he expressed culture as the 'root of everyone', his 'black heritage' from parental background; he also described how the difficulty with mental illness led to an impairment of his identity due to 'not knowing' who he was:

> *"You know something, I still have that same root there you know, because the root of everyone is part of their culture. The root of me is my parent and the root of my parents is their parents, from that same heritage, the black heritage. So my culture is in that black heritage um.... so, when I had my mental health issue, it was all over the place um...I didn't know who I was erm...I didn't know where I was coming from".* (1-1).

This further highlights the importance of culture in identity, and the idea of losing the self as expressed here also connotes losing a sense of control of one's identity, which is an element which may also impact on the externality of LOC. Tim's statement also includes an example of this view of the importance of culture. He describes his culture within the context of music and spirituality, the impact of the type of music he was listening to, which he, in turn, attributes to be part of his culture:

> *"I read the bible most days. I went to meetings, prayer meetings...er..my culture now...oh and the music I was listening to was quite uplifting but some of the words were negative to me it was good but some of the words to me*

> *were negative and that's part of my culture erm....and that affected me"* (FG2).

The expressed view around music, participating in prayer meetings and bible reading also seem to be in line with the predominant view by most of the participants that the culture of spirituality, prayers and listening to music were important parts of their culture as A & C groups. However, the perception that the absence of these aspects of the culture were indicated to have impacted on their view of control over their lives and contributed to the externality in LOC of most of the participants in mental health settings. This is further buttressed by the idea expressed by most of the participants that their culture is a way by which their relationships are directed and guided. An example of this there is Alison's statement in which she described her culture as a means of understanding the world, and a way for her to relate with the services in the context of the 'normal wider community':

> *"So my culture helps me to see the world and understand it around me ummm... in the mental system and to see the normal wider community and I've got to be wise really..."* (1-1).

The idea expressed suggests the importance the participants place on their culture to gain insight into making sense of their experiences with services and gain control of their situation from a position of externality. It also seems to suggest that they see it as a tool to regaining control and leading to internality in their LOC.

An example of the expressed importance of culture in identity by most of the participants is included in Brian's statement in relation to his experience of the services. He described culture in relation to both his 'identity', 'heritage' and 'traditions':

> *"If I lose that culture, I lose my identity...I lose my heritage....I lose my traditions and that's what happened to me in the mental health system when I first went into it, I lost all control of all of that"* (FG1).

A description of losing control of these concepts in his dealing with the mental health system is also an indication of their importance from the perspective of the participants, and in turn suggests that a feeling of losing control over them led to externality in their mental health LOC. Alison also commented on her perception of the importance of her culture by citing historical perspectives in formulating her identity; she also indicated that she continues with practicing her culture from the perspective of hair care and diet:

> *"... I'm from African Black Caribbean um... living in the *** because of the trans- Atlantic race war that really started in the 14th century and I'm the result of that. However, throughout the years my culture has persisted for instance for example I eat Caribbean food which is basically African food more than I eat white English food because I think it's generally better for me. The way we say things and the way we do things are really quite different from English people, although I've been adapted to their culture; their culture is not my culture. For example, my hair.... My hair is strictly Negro hair. I do not perm my hair, but I wash it, I oil it and I plat it up. I also wear lovely head scarves, all different ones because that's also traditional and cultural to my people. That's my identity, and they have to believe it".* (1-1).

By highlighting the differences in culture to express their identity, from historical ambit, it suggests that the participants sought to differentiate the importance of the culture to their ability to control their lives, the absence of which would lead to externality. They also commented that, although their culture was the basis of their identity, the absence of consideration for their culture in their mental health experience was in turn impacting on their perception of control, as they felt that they were not in control of their lives as a result of this phenomenon. An example of the expression of loss is included in Tim's statement in which he expressed that he was seeking to regain his identity lost in the course of his experience with services, and 'finding self':

> *"...and I'm trying to find my identity back and what I do now .... (in an MH charity) is helping me to find myself..."* (FG2).

Another example of the impact of the mental illness experience on the sense of loss of identity and culture, and externality in LOC as a consequence is included in Patrick's statement in which he described 'origin', a sense of loss in his hospital experience, and a feeling of having to 'start again':

> *"I was born in London, but my own origin as someone from Jamaica and what we do is also my culture, that's me... not someone else's identity. Because I lost all that when there was nobody I had to start again, looking for my friends. No family either, it's awful."* (Patrick, 1-1).

This expression of difference in cultures from origin and the place of birth as well as a need to 'start again' seem to suggest that the externality in LOC in mental health is characterised by a loss of control over own life due to feeling a loss of control over identity. It also seems to be in line with the view expressed under the super theme of the level of control-mental illness triggers, in which identity challenges were predominantly identified as being causative to the mental illness trigger. This also suggests that the after-discharge experience is characterised by a continuation of this perception of a loss of identity and culture, and a desire to regain their LOC by regaining and controlling their sense of identity and culture.

The role of culture in identity was also expressed by most of the participants from the context of the role played by shared identity. They expressed that meeting people who shared their identity and culture in their experiences with services played a role in their perception of control (leading to internality in LOC). This was expressed as a result of being able to identify with those people and feeling that they had a common sense of belonging, and peer support with them.

An example of this perspective is contained in Dylan's statement in which he described the possibility of starting a relationship easily with people who has a 'cultural understanding' of people's backgrounds, and benefiting from such relationships:

> *" ....you know, if you meet someone who knows something about you like where you're coming from or your interests yeah....you can strike up a relationship with that person and you can start to trust them in some kind of way and feel that they're very ....ummm...you know, you know that you can alleviate your problems that they might give you an insight into yourself you know... so that a cultural understanding of people's background and of where they are coming from yeah.."* (Dylan, 1-1).

This perspective is buttressed by a statement by Alan in which he cited a hospital experience to highlight the link between shared cultural interests, which led to him being able to 'get on with' some health professionals:

> *"..when someone can click with you, for instance I remember getting into a discussion with some of the night duty ....nurses, about FelaKuti (*a famous African musician) *and ummm... we were talking about FelaKuti.....and ummmm....you know...I related to him and we were talking about FelaKuti and you know I was able to get on with them and different things and you know, little things like that can help you know".* (Alan, 1-1).

He added with another example with the link of this with his response to treatment:

> *"..You know like I met another guy and you know at that time I was on an injection yeah and ... he said to me, he said to me "listen, you're meant to have your injection yeah" and I said "I have; don't want it" and he said to me well......if you don't want it, there's nothing I can do about it. So, I took my injection just because we really started to*

> *communicate, we started to communicate. Yeah, He was a black person and we started to get on and...we started to get on and I just took the injection and that was the last injection I took you know? So, you know.... a person's attitude and the way they relate to you... you know.... I know it.....I know it....everybody"* (Alan, 1-1).

These narrations suggest that relationships were improved between the clients and the health professional due to shared culture and interests. It also indicates that a shared identity can improve relationships and potentially lead to culturally-adapted approaches by health professionals. This could, in turn, lead to internal LOC in the clients, as they are encouraged to perceive that they can take decisions rather than being forced or coerced. An example of this is found in Brian's statement in which he expressed the importance of culture on the clients and their sense of identity. He described a culture that included the use of illicit drugs, music and parties:

> *"The smoking the marijuana, the link with my culture was the music. That's what it was. It was the music I was playing. I used to be a professional musician. I used to play with professional bands, in the music scene, in the black scene in London erm....so that was a big thing for me in them days, that was my music, my culture, the going out, the blues parties, the clubs you know.....going on trips with the band you know. It was all music and food at that time and umm...er er......and that was my culture then."* (FG1).

This quotation suggests that an understanding of the culture and taking into consideration of the tradition and practices may enable the health professionals to recognise and assess the socio-cultural practices and their impact on the health of their clients.

These findings also indicate that the professionals need to gain a greater insight into the individual and group dynamics that operate within the A & C peoples as it relates to them as service users, in order to meet their needs. They also need to understand the cultural implications for mental health and be able to design suitable mental health support based on the information regarding the culture and practices.

3.2. Significance of Family in Culture and LOC

This subtheme contains the responses of the participants to the question as to the extent to which they believed that their culture played a role in their perception of control over their lives. Most participants articulated that their family members were an important aspect of their culture. As a result of this, most related the importance of family to their experience of services; they also expressed that members of their family and their friends were not involved in their treatment or in decisions made towards their welfare. This, in turn, was expressed as leading to their feeling of being without control due to their view that services were ignoring the role played by their family members in their health.

One example of this perception is aptly illustrated in Leonie's statement in which she indicated the importance of her mother to her experience, expressing that she felt that services did not consider the importance of family members to the clients:

> *"It would have been good if my mum was involved, as she used to visit me and bring me food. She is important to me as the only member who cares for me....but it was not so, what can I say? They don't want to know that family is important to us"* (FG1).

Another example is contained in Bianca's statement in which she described the feeling that their trust of the services becomes eroded when they feel that members of their families were not included in decision making, even when the family members make the effort to get involved in the health care process:

> *"......how they've been treated so the trust is not there. They may see how their friends or family and they might have tried to get involved in their care of their loved ones and care and not being welcome or their point of view not taken*

into account or umm.... Involved in the decision-making process so they don't see them necessarily as people that want to work with them. They just see that these people have power over them, and nobody wants to be controlled or have power umm... have other people have power over them..." (Bianca, 1-1).

This viewpoint seems to indicate that as the inclusion of members of their families was an indication that their opinions were considered and that they had some form of control due to family involvement, and an internality in LOC as a consequence; the absence of this ability to exert influence via the involvement of their family members and friends seem to suggest that it has resulted in externality in their LOC that has been expressed.

In highlighting the importance of the role of family members and relatives, it was also expressed that the presence of family members in hospital settings acted as a protective factor for the way they received treatment and the extent to which their concerns were addressed. This highlights the role of family members as an important support against a powerful and sometimes coercive system. One example of this perception was articulated by a participant who felt that their opinions were being ignored, especially when their family members were not around. Bianca pointed out that her expressed needs were being brushed 'under the carpet', culminating in her feeling that the absence of family and friends meant that she was at the mercy of services, and that 'they can do with you what they want'. Also, by referring to such an experience as 'additional trauma', she explained that she felt that such experience would not be applicable to white patients:

"...do you know because I was in that situation and if you tried to express that you are feeling a certain way they would just try and brush it under the carpet. Your voice was no longer valid. Especially when you didn't have your friends or relative around you so basically, they can do with you what they want. If you had a qualm, then it would be

> *your word against theirs. I didn't feel like the white patients had to deal with this additional trauma".* (Bianca, 1-1).

This viewpoint seems to suggest that many patients may be so disaffected as a result of their perception that they lack control over their experiences or their lives with services to the extent that they felt that having members of their families and friends around would offer them some sort of support or 'protection' of their rights to be heard. This further indicates that their LOC would be external in this respect as a result of a feeling of a need to get further support to help them gain control which they perceived to have been lost.

This is further illustrated in the views expressed by most participants in which they expressed the perception of the importance of family members' willingness to engage in the health care process, as being highly important in leading to positive response of the healthcare professionals. An example of this view is contained in Carla's statement in which she indicated that the willingness of family members and close friends in the clients' experience with services are likely to make the clients feel that their involvement will reduce the likelihood of them experiencing 'something going wrong' or being 'taken advantage of':

> *"Well if there's support around and family and closer friends are willing to engage, I think the professionals should show the willingness to involve them so ... let the patient feel like they have somebody looking over their shoulder to make sure or to try and reduce the likelihood of something going wrong or them being taken advantage of..."* (Carla, FG2).

This also seems to indicate that the participants felt that they need the input of their family members and close friends to support them and act as advocates on their behalf to allay their fears of poor experience or wrong doing in their experiences. This also is an indication of externality in LOC, as they seem to need someone to protect their rights and welfare, which they feel is likely to be compromised without the family and friends' involvement.

Another perspective within this perception of the lack of acknowledgement of the role of family members and the need to engage with them by professionals, which, in turn, plays a role in the feeling of lack of control (externality in LOC) was expressed by most participants from the parlance of what they perceived as the way each party (the family members and the health professionals) sees their relationship in relation to the mental health experiences of the clients. It is largely viewed by the participants that the family members see themselves as not being considered by the health professionals as an integral part of the mental health experiences of their family member who is in hospital, while the health professionals consider themselves to be in control of decisions as they oversaw caring for the patient. An example of this view is contained in a statement by Bianca, in which she cited that a barrier exists between the psychiatrist and family members (whom she referred to as carers) - in which the family members feel that the psychiatrists were ignoring them and the psychiatrists query the right of the family member to be involved in what they termed as they are being 'in charge' of:

> *".... but invariably again, there is a barrier between the psychiatrist and the other carers. The carers don't' feel like the psychiatrists are listening to them and the psychiatrists are probably thinking "well I'm the psychiatrist, I know what I'm doing, who are you to tell me what to do? you know, I'm in charge of your patient, the patient is under my care and they need to do what I say"..."* (Bianca, 1-1).

This viewpoint also indicates that the majority of the participants were trying to make sense of the possible reason behind a factor that contributes to their feeling a lack of control (external LOC), in their mental health experiences with services due to a lack of involvement of their family members and close friends. It indicates also that their LOC has become external to the extent that they are able to explain their own perspective of the possible reason for which they were unable to exert any influence on their experience through the involvement of their family members and friends.

3.3. Perception That Their Culture Was Being Ignored in Respect of Diet and Other Support for Self-Care in Hospitals

This subtheme also contains another set of issues relating to the perception of the study participants to the relationship between their experiences with services and their culture. In response to the question regarding if they felt that culture played a role in their experience with services, the majority of the participants indicated that their culture was not considered in their experience in hospital by the mental health services and professionals. It was observed that most of the responses relating to culture were highly centred on issues of dietary requirements and other self-care including skin care provisions, which majority of the participants felt strongly about, as they stressed that their cultural needs as A & C groups were ignored. An example of this view is included in Stella's statement in which she expressed that culture could not be expected to be in the forefront of expectation whilst an inpatient in hospital (infirmary), expressing that 'food is part of someone's culture', and some elements of finality that 'no matter how much you're asking and you beg'; to indicate an element of frustration that culturally specific dietary requirements like 'yam dumpling and banana' were not met for A & C groups by services.

> *"With being in.....in, in in in....an infirmary you can't necessarily put culture first and that's a fact because number one you're not going to get yam dumplings and banana in your food. You're not and no matter how much you're asking, and you beg and you please, you're not going to get that as a meal full stop. You're either going to get frozen food that's been in the freezer for how long no one knows, and food is part of someone's culture and strength definitely. So, if someone is messing with your food and messing with your health and messing with your culture and tampering with things so, it's just to better yourself in the way you know that you can. So, you can ask them for halal food, fine; they'll still stigmatise you, they'll still label you, they'll still stigmatise you whatever..."* (Stella, 1-1)

The notion of 'messing with your food' expressed within the context of messing with 'health' and 'culture' expressed here suggests that there is an intersection between the three concepts of diet, health and culture. The externality in mental health LOC is also highlighted in the low expectation expressed by the participants that their culture that is important to them cannot be 'put first' in their mental health experiences. The notion also expressed as 'they still stigmatise you' also suggests that there is a potential reluctance to express one's desire for culturally based diet, for fear of negative consequences, including a feeling of being given a 'label' in the hospital setting. This fear of expressing need is also an indication of externality in LOC, as the individual concerned may choose not to engage or expressing their view as they deem fit, as they are likely to feel that it will not bring any positive outcome but may lead to even worse situations for them. Another example of this view is included in Melanie's statement in which she expressed some sarcasm regarding a lack of care for her cultural needs for skin care, hair care and food. She refers to having dry skin, not being provided 'Caribbean food', and not receiving care for her hair:

> *"No, I'm a Caribbean, they never provided Caribbean food for me, (laughs) you must be joking. I have Negro skin, my skin got very dry. Did they provide oil and cream for my skin? No! So the food in hospital was English food, that horrible mushed up rubbish (laughs). Did they provide for my hair, did they say oh once a week somebody will come by and oil and cream my hair and comb it and plat it up for me? No, I looked like a ragamuffin, thank you very much. No!" (Melanie,* FG2).

Gerald's statement also included the expressed importance of food in their culture, the type of food he requires, and he also expressed trying to 'get my old culture back':

> *"My culture is yam, banana, swordfish…all the different food because food is part of culture…..Some people have lost their culture and go into a different kind of culture*

> *whereas I'm trying to get my old culture back...with the culture that I'm already in, in the mental health system..."* (Gerald, 1-1)

The expression of having 'English food' and lacking the cultural food also suggests that the participants' cultural preferences were not being considered. In addition, as hair and skin care were also considered as important to the A & C groups, the lack of support for these needs as expressed by Carla above also indicates that the externality in their LOC might have originated from their perception that they had no control over their food and self-care needs. Another example of this dynamic is included in Noella's statement in which she referred to her ward visiting experience as a peer support client. She mentioned that care could be improved for BME groups from paying attention to their diet:

> *"How could they improve it? By the way that they care for them, by the food that they give them...."* (1-1).

In relating food to care in addition to observing that clients are not provided the cultural food 'that they're are used to', she also suggested that professionals need to 'interact' more with their clients and conduct surveys regarding their needs:

> *"They haven't got the foods that BME people require or that they're used to, they haven't; not really. Care, food, a survey.* And that: *"They need to do a survey. Again, they need to interact with them more, they need training"*. (1-1).

Another example of the view of a lack of culturally-focused care regarding food was expressed in Brian's statement in which he described the involvement of his family members in solving the food problem:

> *"I never used to get my own food... like my own culture food, my parents had to cook it and bring it up on a Sunday. If it wasn't for that meal, I'd probably be lost within the mental health system"*. (FG1)

The expression by Brian of not getting his 'own food' here and relying on his parents suggests externality in LOC in a lack of control over the type of food he received from services, which necessitated him taking advantage of the option open to him via support from his family. The expression of the likelihood of being 'lost within the mental health system' if the participant did not receive support from the parents also indicates not only the importance placed on culturally-focused food by the participants but also indicates a sense of helplessness (externality) could have been enhanced to detrimental effect without the family support. Alan's statement also contains an example of this view that the foods needed by clients of BME origin are not provided. He cites examples of swordfish, dumpling and curry goat, which are not available for the groups, stating also that 'your culture can be affected by the foods that you eat':

> *"...on the ward when they serve food it doesn't have the kind of food that people from certain black cultures eat and that's also a negative point....a negative point for someone who's got mental problems because you could be on the ward and want to eat swordfish or dumpling or curry goat or patties and they're the kinds of foods they don't necessarily have. Sometimes your culture can be affected by the foods that you eat and em...being in the mental health system they don't give you those things to eat on the ward you know".* (1-1).

This view is also included in Patrick's statement, giving examples of soup, rice and beans for African groups which he states are not available in the hospitals as 'they don't cook it there':

> *"You eat you know, how you eat as a black person, a Caribbean person from my perspective or if you're African, you eat soup or beans and that can be another issue that they might not have those kinds of foods for people who are BME, you know who eat those kinds of foods regularly like rice and beans chicken and stuff like that and they don't cook it there".* (FG1).

These views are indicators that the food provided to the clients from the A & C populations contrast with their cultural dietary needs. It also connotes a perception that the participants had no control over the food they were given but had to rely on the support of their family members who were able to supply them such meals to them in hospital. This is also an element of externality in their LOC in mental health settings, as they perceived that they had no control over this aspect of their cultures. This externality also seems to be highlighted as it has been generally stated by the majority of the participants that food is an integral part of their culture, which is integral to their identity as groups of the A & C backgrounds. Another example of this view is contained in Leonie's statement in which she described the importance of culture to the way she takes care of her hair, resorting to plaiting rather than 'perming', and also described having to revert to her 'Caribbean African food' after hospitalisation, for health reasons:

> *"...Well for me, for myself, culture played a great important part. It was also looking in the mirror, and thinking yeah, I am a Black woman, I am going to tie my head. That was a big part of it. Not only that, my mother died, and I thought, you know what, my mother left me all these beautiful head scarfs and I have beautiful, Negro, African hair and I stopped going to the hair dressers and getting all the perming crap. It cost me a lot of money and it didn't do me any good. Ahm....so I decided to wash my hair, comb it and plait it and it's beautiful and I would just wear my head scarf. And looking after myself nutrition wise, I reverted back to eating my Caribbean African food, which I found out was better for me because I was Diabetic as well"* (FG1).

The expressed experience of 'looking at the mirror', reverting in diet and making other changes regarding hair care suggests post-discharge action which demonstrates internality in LOC. It also suggests that although there were experiences of externality in LOC during hospital stay due to expressed inability to control the services they received in terms of hair, food and skin care, efforts are being made by the participants after discharge to regain control over their lives by making decisions to care for their hair in ways that were not available for them whilst in hospital.

3.4. Low Perception of African and Caribbean Culture by Mental Health Services

This subtheme contains an element of the majority of the participants' answers to the question regarding the extent to which they perceived that culture played a role in their mental health experiences- the view regarding the opinion, attitude and judgement of health professionals in relation to the culture of A & C groups in services. Most of the responses were expressed from the ambit of a notion that the health professionals have a low opinion of the culture of A & C groups. This notion was also expressed by most of the participants as being responsible for what they have expressed as inequality in treatment on account of culture in their mental health experiences, and externality in their LOC. This suggests a perception of conscious or unconscious bias and discrimination on account of culture as well as a feeling that the professionals regard their culture as inferior. They also mostly expressed the view that they felt strongly that they had no control over their mental health experiences due to what they perceived as inequality in treatment which emanated from a lack of consideration for their culture by the health professionals, which they attribute to low preconception, prejudice and prejudgement of their cultures as Black people.

These concerns expressed could be considered as having been influenced by their mental health challenges. However, as these misgivings regarding their culture were strongly articulated by most of the participants in the context of their hospital experiences some years after they had been discharged, it suggests that these concerns may have some strong merits and are may not be likely to have been influenced by symptoms of paranoia or delusion. It was also expressed by most participants that they experienced inequality in the way they were treated due to their ethnic origin as A & C groups; most of these experiences were also expressed in relation to their interactions with the psychiatrists, whom they perceive as being highly unaware of the need to consider their intrinsic cultural norms and customs in their approaches to the clients. It also includes the perceived power of the psychiatrists and other health professionals which the participants suggested impacted on their perception of control and externality in LOC. This perception of power was also expressed within the context of perceived imbalance due to a perceived notion that the psychiatrists regard the A & C clients to be of lower cultural, socio-economic and educational status, which they, in turn, expressed as a factor that impacted on their perception of control, leading to their externality in LOC in their mental health experiences.

Within the context of a lack of control on account of culture, one example of this perception included the expression of feeling powerless, not valued, due to a feeling of being treated differently as persons of A & C culture, which impacted on their recovery. An example of this view is indicated in Mary's statement; she expressed feeling a 'cultural barrier' and not 'feeling valued', which impacted negatively on her mental health:

> *"...as a person of erm...BME origin I did feel quite powerless because even though I submitted voluntarily erm.... a lot of my carers* (professionals) *were not of the same culture as myself. I did feel that there was erm.... a cultural barrier and I didn't feel, I didn't feel valued. I just felt like.... very demoralised which actually resulted in my mental health deteriorating. Ummm....so I think it wasn't really from my perspective, it was how people perceived me as an individual and that I was just a mad person and they didn't value me as an individual which I believe had a detrimental effect on my recovery, sorry".* (Mary, 1-1)

The expression of not feeling valued as an individual by professionals of different culture on account of being a Black person who is 'mad' suggests an indicator for externality in LOC, particularly as it was expressed as having led to deterioration in mental health of the individual and their recovery. It also suggests that the participants relate their recovery to their LOC, which, in turn, is inherent in their ability to influence decisions made regarding their health. Another example of this perception of inequality on account of culture and consequent impact on their feeling of lack of control included a participant's description of a perceived preferential treatment on cultural difference basis in a hospital experience:

> *"Well unfortunately in this ward a lot of us were black so we couldn't really differentiate between that ermmm...most of us were black. There was still a hand full of white folks there and still they were given preferential treatment. Even how you'd speak to people regardless of whether they are ill or not, they still deserve a standard of respect. I just felt that I was well enough to see that there was a difference in how we were treated."* (FG2).

A feeling of being disrespected as well as observing other people being 'given preferential treatment' on account of cultural differences also suggests that these experiences are likely to lead to externality in LOC of the individuals who perceive such partiality. Another example of this perception is contained in a description of an experience of being treated with aggression and lack of care as follows:

> *"Well, depending on how it's not necessarily what people say, it's how they say it. I remember a few times where they'd offer me to maybe go for dinner...it's the way they say it. It was very aggressive, it was very uncaring, it was very unwelcoming and so that didn't have a positive effect on my recovery either"*. (1-1)

Within this perception of inequality on account of culture was also included the expression by many participants of feeling being treated as someone of less value by services' professionals. An example of this view is contained in Alison's statement in which she referred to her perception of the way she was treated by the health professionals was without due consideration for her personal professional status or intelligence before becoming unwell. She referred to being 'just seen' as mentally ill black person, and being of 'no value':

> *"...regardless of the fact that it doesn't necessarily matter what profession you are you're all ...or how intelligent you were when you were well ermmm you are all just seen as mentally ill black people. It's almost like you have no value"* (Allison, 1-1).

This seems to indicate that the participants perceive that the health professionals from the mainstream population belittle their clients from the A & C populations on account of their mental illness. This also suggests that the clients perceive that the professionals practice stigma and discrimination against the clients on account of their mental health challenges. This may also indicate that the LOC of the participants are external as a result of this perception that health professionals see Black clients as being of lower value due to their mental illness. This may also exacerbate the perception that they may feel that there would be no need to try to exert any influence on their experience, as the other party who is the health professional deem them to be less intelligent and of less value, are therefore likely to ignore them and their views, and are also likely to not ask them for their opinions regarding their health. This may further lead to externality in LOC.

Another example of this perception includes a feeling of being treated with a lack of respect in the approaches was also cited by Mary, who expressed that she felt that it was necessary not to be treated as 'kicking a dog when it is down':

> *"...We're all ill but still yes we're all here to get better but you should still treat us with the respect that you would have given if we were well. You do not use that as the opportunity to just, excuse the pun but kick a dog when they're down..."* (1-1)

This view of being 'down' may also suggest a feeling of a lack of power or control as a result of the mental illness experience, also an indication for externality in LOC. A feeling expressed also by the participants that they would have been treated with more respect if they had not been ill also suggesting that they felt that their right to be respected has been demeaned by the professionals due to their illness experience.

In addition, within this perception of unequal treatment by health professionals due to low view of the culture of A & C clients, the majority of the participants also raised the role played by the difference in culture and gender between them and the health care professionals, which suggests that this may have impacted on their ability to engage with the professional, and ultimately their perception of control in relation to their experience of service. An example below included the perception of unsatisfactory care experience expressed due to cultural and gender differences in the belief by the participants that white male psychiatrists would not be able to identify with the A & C women on their mental health issues. This was expressed by Bianca:

> *"Well I don't' really think he could identify with me because he's not black and he's not a woman. So whether it was the fact he wasn't black and that played the main part in him not being able to identify with me or whether it was the fact that I was a woman it's difficult to differentiate, I don't know but all I do know is that I didn't get the care that I felt that I should have received".* (Bianca, 1-1).

This suggests that there is an intersectionality of gender, ethnicity and culture and the experiences by A & C clients with services, which in turn contribute to externality in the LOC of the A & C clients.

Another example of the issue of culture was expressed in a statement by Carla in the context of understanding of the personal situations, including migration and relationship issues that may affect the clients:

> *"Because they are being misunderstood, they're being misunderstood because their needs are not being met; their cultural needs are not being met...they are not understanding where they've come from. I mean they could*

have come from a war-torn country. English mightn't be their first language, simple little things even; that they don't look at...that they overlook. You know, their family dynamics, just different things; marital breakdowns.... anything". (Carla, FG2).

Another example included expressions of this perception of inequality in hospital experiences, feeling of perceived experience of disrespect and discrimination on account of culture, especially in the way complaints were perceived to not be attended to but dismissed. One participant described this view as having led to perpetuating the perception of 'a lot more discrimination' and consequent loss of control:

"Well when I was being looked after by white nurses I just felt that they saw me as nothing and just really disrespected me and because I was in that position I couldn't' really defend myself and if I were to raise a complaint they would just say "oh she's mad, she doesn't know what she's talking about" so you face a lot more discrimination umm...when you were being cared for by white professionals". (Jane, FG1).

Another participant described an experience in which they perceived that they were being ignored by the healthcare professionals due to the difference in culture, their description of reaction to this perception, referred to as 'rebelling', which in turn resulted in being physically restrained by the professionals:

"Once I've been er.....cornered off erm.....really been cornered off and I didn't understand because I just went into my room to sleep and one of the nurses wouldn't open the door at all. I was in there for half an hour and it was like I was being ignored so um...they just wouldn't let me go and rest, they said no; so I rebelled and kicked the door which was a door...a magnetised door and the door was like totally close and it needed a buzzer to open it like it was a magnet

> *basically. That was the only way that I got their attention because then decided to obviously push the button. They obviously thought I was too calm without drugs. So I kicked the door, kicked the door, kicked the door and then they came out and then they all started to restrain me. I have no idea what they did to me but anyway then I slept, and I slept and I slept".* (Trish, FG2).

The expression of feeling ignored for about half an hour due to perceived cultural differences as well as going through the experience of having to express one's frustration is an indication of rebelling against what is perceived as external control against which one has no control over. This scenario also represents a protest perceived external LOC in which the participant quoted tried to exercise some form of control, albeit to negative consequences.

Many participants also stated that they felt that they were treated without sympathy due to their culture. An example of this perception is contained in Alan's statement in which he cited an example in which he made a complaint regarding being treated without consideration, describing his experience as 'very cold and unsympathetic':

> *"Well I wrote a letter of complaint about this doctor and about the treatment and I had here and I explained how this guy hadn't listened to me and I had even written him a 6 page letter of how ill I was and I hadn't even mentioned race or anything in it, but he happened to be a European doctor and immediately I didn't mention race of colour it was a racist thing but I was just outlining the situation and the way he treated me was very cold and very unsympathetic, he treated me in that way ...".*(1-1)

Alan also used this experience to express the perceived lack of 'voice' experienced by mental health clients when they feel that they were treated without sympathy by health care professionals:

> *"...and we are talking about many people with schizophrenia without a voice. They can't speak up for themselves and because they meet up with someone who is unsympathetic to them.... because you never know, you never know who you're meeting. That's reality. You don't know who you're meeting in this society. Just because they say they are this or they're that that doesn't mean they are fully rounded persons or that they are sympathetic or. I mean, this guy showed me no care whatsoever. It really did make me ill. I mean, I had the worst nightmares when I was dealing with him. That's all I can say".* (1-1)

The perceived use of power by Psychiatrists also featured within the context of the expressed feelings of many of the participants that the culture of the A & C groups was not considered while dealing with them. Most participants discussed their perception that the power exercised by the psychiatrist was directed by the role played by differences in culture between them as clients and the psychiatrist as a professional who has power and authority. For example, Jane described an inability to be 'in tune' with her psychiatrist due to this difference in culture, and asserted that there would have been a difference in 'dialogue' and outcome if she had come from Caucasian background:

> *"... perhaps if I had been a British Caucasian, I would have been more in tune to the (Caucasian) professional that was sitting in front of me and it possibly could have been an easier dialogue than it was".* (FG1)

This opinion was also expressed by Bianca that the difference in culture also plays a role in the perception of the psychiatrist, their opinion and judgement made by them over the behaviours and characteristics of the clients from the community, due to what they perceived as a lack of cultural awareness:

> *"...that is based on somebody's perception and opinion so that's usually the psychiatrist erm...his or her opinion or perspective and they may not be culturally aware of*

different diversities and so on. So, their opinion of erratic behaviour may just be annoyance of some kind, just a way that particular people express themselves" (Bianca, 1-1)

Bianca also articulated that as a result of this, clients also need to focus on responding to this issue even when they are unwell:

> *"So you have to try, even though you're not well and you have to try and always remember that the person sitting opposite you; doesn't necessarily know you and doesn't know where you're coming from. They don't know your behavioural characteristics but yet they are in a position of authority and in control of whether you are admitted or prescribed certain medications and.....in order for you to be......in order for you to get through the system sometimes you have to go along with it"* (Bianca, 1-1).

It was also expressed by Jane that it was necessary for the clients from the community to manage their responses to the actions of the health care professionals due to their perception of the power the latter exert:

> *"Well again because my grandma used to say that we hold the blade and they hold the handle, even because they are in control of what you are prescribed and how you can be perceived by other professionals within the multidisciplinary team; you still have to be careful of how you behave because of stereotypes associated with BME community".* (Jane, FG1)

The perceived impression of the professionals regarding the A & C clients due to the cultural factors was also expressed by most participants in the context of perceived fear of Black clients by the professionals. For example, Dwayne described this perception of fear due to lack of understanding of the culture leads to a desire to control, medication and sedation:

> *"Ummmm but again I can understand the fear because when you're unwell and you can appear very umm.... erratic in your behaviour and they don't understand you and so when you don't understand something, you just want to control it. You just want to encage it so that is one of the few powers if you want to put it, that the mental health services have over....when dealing with black people. i.e....giving them as much medication as you can give them to sedate them. So that they're no longer a threat to you or themselves or anybody else but that may not necessarily be the right thing to do".* (1-1).

This expression of fear of violence and aggression was also perceived as indicative of the feeling of suspicion by the professionals that most participants believed led to being subjected to readmissions. An example of this perception was described by Ryan when he illustrated that professionals visited his home and described 'sectioning' in the context of him being 'locked up' due to suspicion of murder or stealing:

> *"...to me that more than likely they will come back to your house and section you again, they always turn up and it's a knock on the door with the team, they just open the door and say, 'Mr. Xxx, we think you're planning to do murders, that's it and we think you're planning to murder people and you're planning to steal and blah blah and I tried to contest it and they just called the doctor and locked me up and I can't do anything about it. So, I think that because of the culture that I come from that's what affects it you know, affects the way they treat you and that's how it was for me anyway"* (Ryan, 1-1).

The concern illustrated in this example relates to being placed under some specific sections of the MHA (2007), including Sections 2, 3 and the Section 17a (Supervised Community Treatment (SCT). The participants perceive that they are being 'sectioned' as a result of suspicion of them as Black groups. This further corroborates what obtains in literature to the effect that the notion of dangerousness of A & C groups (Keating, 2012; Edge, 2013) places them to be vulnerable to being sectioned and other coercive practices at a higher rate than people of the mainstream cultures.

Another example of the perception of existence of fear of the Black people by the professionals due to a lack of understanding of culture was expressed in the description of an episode by Mary, where the health professionals mistook her action to wipe off the sand on her footwear (slippers) by hitting them on the wall for aggression which led to a decision to section her:

> *"Would you say this is culture, before when I ... there was a doctor and a CPN at my house, I had my slippers on and they said you need to take those off and so I took my slippers off and I hit them against the wall to get the dust off before I put them in the cupboard. She went "right, you're sectioned, you're definitely sectioned now". I said "what?"* (Mary, 1-1).

Another example of this perception is contained in Ryan's expression that the fear of A & C clients by professionals led to the latter's view that it was necessary to control their Black clients by physical restraint or use of drugs, without considering if some factors such as experience of environmental racism could have impacted on their behaviours:

> *"Because of the way that they approach them, that could be one thing. It could just be their life experiences of growing up in this environment, where they've had to experience racism in schools umm in the media they're always portrayed as bad or unsavoury people so it could well be how the doctor is conditioned to see black patients and they're fearful of them and they want to control them. You either control them through physical restraint or you control them through drugs"* (Ryan, 1-1).

What most of the participants perceived should be the behavioural response of the clients as a result of this perceived fear was also expressed by Alison to include the perceived need to avoid creating a wrong impression of appearing aggressive or violent to avoid being 'sedated':

> *"You have to make sure you don't give the wrong impression, that you're not appearing to be aggressive or appearing to be violent because I believe that there's a fear with....when treating with people of this community and invariably we are the ones that tend to be sedated more readily or given high doses than many of our white counterparts"* (Alison, 1-1).

This perception expressed in the context of the perceived need for the Black clients to approach the professionals in a specific way in the belief that the latter already perceived a fear of the existence of aggression and uncooperative attitude dominated the position of most of the participants. In an example of these expressions, one participant likened going to the professionals to applying for employment, mentioning that approaching the professionals 'in a specific manner' was likely to make their and views 'more palatable' and result in positive outcomes for the Black client:

> *"Well I think although we have as black people or BME people have valuable things to say, because of ; I know it seems unfair but because of other communities perception of us we need to know how to approach umm... approach these professionals because we have to believe that they may have a fear there already of black people being aggressive or you know ummmm not being particularly cooperative...so we need to know how to for example if you go for a job you show your best face so basically you need to know how best to get what you want from the psychiatrist by approaching them in a specific manner to make it more palatable for them to accept what you're saying or take on board your opinion. It might now mean*

> *that they agree with your opinion but at later if they're listening to you, you're more likely to get the response that you want"* (Tim, FG2).

The expressed need for the Black client to only express their views in ways that would be considered acceptable by the professionals suggests that there is a likelihood that the A & C client may feel that they had no control over their relationship with the professionals (externality in the LOC). It also suggests that the clients were likely to avoid going to the professional for support, as they were not likely to be agreeable to telling the professionals what they wanted to hear or in ways they want to be approached.

The importance of approaching the professionals in specific ways was also expressed in the context of the likelihood that perceived aggression or being uncooperative goes on the clients' medical files by the professionals. This, in turn, is perceived to be perpetuating the impression of the clients' behaviour and the likelihood of this perception to lead to more negative reactions by other professionals and poor treatment outcome:

> *"Well it's on your record so therefore, providing it's on your record other professionals will see this information and....because...this information is stored.... other professionals will see this information and perhaps come to an opinion about you without really knowing you without knowing the reason behind it. Everybody knows that appointments are time restricted and so not every doctor, or not every psychiatrist is going to be able to go in depth into why you behaved in a particular way at a particular time. They are just going to read the notes and assume based on a previous experience which may not necessarily be your overall personality".* (Bianca, 1-1).

Another example of this perception was contained in a description by another participant in the context of the fear of services from the perspective of Black people, 'the circles of fear', the stories they hear from other Black people regarding negative experience of services, which, in turn, is perceived to make them avoid seeking help. This was also expressed in the parlance of being avoided by fellow A & C friends for engaging with the services:

> *"Another thing about the fear is when, that person.... I'm not really sure that he's not well or he's got mental health problems. Why don't you tell him what happens? In the mental health system, he might not want to get treatment that's what happens to black people. Once they hear it, they fear it. Breaking the circle, breaking the circle of fear. Some of them don't want to get treatment or be admitted because of the stories they hear about being black in the mental health system so instead they stay away from it. When they see someone, who's been through it and they say "what's it like?" "Don't go in man! They're going to get you, they're going to inject you". But that's just what happens, that's how it works".* (Patrick, FG1).

The expression of 'breaking the circles of fear' highlights the importance placed by the participant to the observed challenges that impact on the reluctance of clients from A & C backgrounds to seek help for mental health challenges. This is also an indication of externality in LOC, as it suggests that the expressed fear of services, fear of being injected, and leading to staying away from services stem from the perception that they will not have control over the decisions made about them by services. It also indicates that the negative experiences and stories regarding those experiences were likely to reinforce negative perceptions. The idea of staying away may also be indicative of a desire for self-preservation, which is a form of internality in LOC.

Another example of the expression of this perception of fear was highlighted in a statement by Dylan, who used his own experience as an example in expressing that the avoidance of services due to fear could lead to further deterioration, and being 'hard to come out of the mental health system':

> *"The problem is with the BME we leave it too long to get treatment, they leave it too long because they fear it. They don't want to go into hospital and that's when your episodes get worse and that's when you tend to call for help and that what it was in my case and by that time it's blown out and the mental health is there and it's hard to come out of the mental health system"*. (Dylan, 1-1).

The perceived fear was also expressed by most participants as impacting on their confidence. An example of this perception is included in expression of lacking confidence, being 'nervy' and fear of psychiatrist, and in which one of the participants also expressed that this feeling could only 'fade' with experience:

> *"At first, I was very nervy, I wasn't confident at all. I was always in fear of the psychologist (psychiatrist) because I did never believe what they could tell you um...about yourself, about you I think the fear and distrust thing.... that kind of thing only really.... really fades with kind of with experience and erm...exposure really"*. (Leonie, FG1).

The expression of 'fear and distrust' in the above quote also suggests externality in LOC which impacts on the relationship between the clients and the psychiatrist. The responses of most participants in relation to the role they perceived culture played in their mental health experience also contained a high level of expressed link between the role played by a lack of consideration of their culture as A & C groups by the psychiatrists and their perception that there was an existence of lower cultural status, educational and socio-economic status. This link was, in turn, perceived by most participants as contributory to the perceived power that has been attributed to the psychiatrists from their perspectives, which in consequent led to their notion of having no power as clients in their dealing with the psychiatrist (externality in LOC). It was also highlighted by majority of the participants that the psychiatrist was operating from a comparatively stronger power base which was also influenced by the psychiatrists' perception that the groups of A & C ethnic extractions were of inferior culture, education and socio-economic status. An example of the expression of unequal balance of power is contained in Noella's statement:

> *"... as a black person I felt suppressed and so therefore if I feel suppressed in that situation then...the footing is not equal.... it's not ..it's ...it's him more than me but the base line isn't the same. He's a Psychiatrist and I'm a ...service user. That's the end of it, there's no, there's no... equal balance"* (Noella, 1-1).

The expression of feeling 'suppressed' and its likely impact on the relationship between the clients and the psychiatrist is also a suggestion of the existence of externality in the mental health LOC of the clients. This is since a feeling of suppression is indicated to end in feeling that one's opinion or view is likely to be ignored to the extent that one feels 'suppressed'. An example of this perception of powerlessness due to lower educational status and comparative skill difference as factors contributory to the perception of power imbalance between the A & C clients and the psychiatrist was also expressed in relation to the observation by most participants that the psychiatrists were mostly from white backgrounds. This includes the expression of 'limited education', having to 'go along' with the psychiatrist's decision, and not being able to 'argue' any difference in opinion, as expressed by Alison.

> *"Your culture plays a role in it because at the end of the day the professional in front of you is a white Caucasian who has the power to prescribe any medication he or she likes. Me in my limited education in medical.... you know, medicines and the body and anatomy and the brain um......because I haven't been blessed with that skill; I have to take that psychiatrists word for it. So, I feel that with my limited knowledge I feel like I have to go along with him or her because...where's my argument? I have to go along because I can't' stop taking it, the only thing I can argue is "Doctor that made me feel...." But I couldn't argue "I'm not*

> *taking it because...." I have to just go along and come back to him or her, that's the only choice I have in the matter because I'm not of the intellect to prescribe which medicine to prescribe myself".* (Alison, 1-1)

The perceived lower socioeconomic, educational background, culture, and 'intellect' and the consequent influence on the perception of power were also expressed by most participants. This includes statements relating to perceived low socio-economic status of parents. An example of this view is contained in Brain's statement in which he described the status of Caribbean parents as not 'coming from that direction' of sending their children to 'the best school', 'best education' and qualifications:

> *"....... because at the end of the day, I wasn't sent to the best schools in London because my parents didn't.... didn't...they weren't ...they weren't coming from that direction. They weren't about sending you to the best school in London, for you to have the best education so you could graduate with all these qualifications. To know about these particular aspects, to know about the body and so on and so forth because when I was going to school, I don't know anybody that was of that intellect, I didn't know anybody".* (FG1).

He further illustrated the social inequalities by citing the parents' working hours, the children 'trying to get by', in comparison to the parents of the Caucasian counterparts who he perceived invested in their children's education; which, in turn, led to a level of inequality and reliance on the Caucasian people with higher educational background:

> *"We were all just trying to get by, our parents were working 8 till 4, 7 till 3 or 7 till 6 sometimes you know, just to be able to get through your school work was a struggle so you then rely on the Caucasian white professional because they're parents invested in things like that. So, I think your*

education does have a part to do with it, your background. Your culture does have a part to do with it because if you're not blessed with that hindsight, how would your child ever achieve more than you?" (Brian FG1).

This perception was also attributed to prejudgment by the health professionals, which, in turn, was perceived as having led to a feeling of lack of control by the Black clients. Alison statement regarding her perception that the Caucasian professional 'knew' that 'a lot of black people ...were not of the intellect as themselves'; the parents' working background, 'Oh, father is a trainman, mother's a cook' to express that the psychiatrist was likely to have prejudged the clients in their treatment approaches:

"Because he knew or she (Psychiatrist) knew that. I was not of the same intellect. They knew. Most professionals that are Caucasian know that... a lot of black people, I'm not saying all because it's not all in my case they knew that I was not of the intellect as themselves. They knew that I was from a working class, black parentage so on and so forth. Because all these questions are asked of you when you're admitted and when you're put under the CMHT and when you're assessed. So, they know your background and they know where you're coming from. Oh, father is a trainman, mother's a cook or whatever". (1-1).

It was also expressed that the perceived prejudgment has an influence in the treatment by the health care professional from the white background, as included in Alison's further expression:

"So, they know, there's a prejudgment in their mind that he or she isn't going to know that much at the end of the day because he or she is just......another young black girl; you know what I mean. I think that's really an influence". (Alison, 1-1).

This suggests that the supposed influence would have negatively impacted on clients' sense of control, thereby leading to have a feeling of externality - the perception that decisions and ultimately control of the mental health experience were not in their hands but in those of the professionals.

Another example of the perceived 'prejudgment' and the link to power and control was surmised to have been demonstrated in what majority of the participants expressed as 'preconceived ideas', body language in speech, eye contact and other indicators in interactions with the professionals This is further expressed by the participants as indicative of how they perceived that power and control are exercised. An example of this view was in the statement by Noella:

> *"I think that people have pre-conceived ideas; I think we all do. We have pre-conceived ideas. The way a person greets you, the way a person speaks to you, the way a person has..body language..eye contact and so on and so forth. They all play, they all play a factor in how you respond to that person. If you're picking up a feeling of anything then obviously it manifests itself because .... that's how you feel I mean...no one can take away how you feel. Because at the end of the day they ...they.... have control over....they have control over....you. well me....don't they?. If they have power, they have control. Power and control work together, I believe so because if you have control then you must have power"*. (1-1).

The perception of lower cultural status was also expressed by most participants as having originated from historical and cultural norms. This was expressed as a factor which, in turn, is perceived to be contributory to the clients' externality in not challenging any unsatisfactory status quo in their mental health experiences, due to a feeling of a lack of control. For example, it was cited by Jane that Black people were normalised to always follow the rules in order not to 'stand out', 'draw attention' to themselves, which in turn contribute to a feeling of having 'no choice' and having to 'go with it' when they perceive that they were not being treated right:

> *"...black people have always been told, well from my experience and from ancestral experience; have always been told to follow the rules. Don't stand out, don't draw attention to yourself so therefore culture does play a big part in it because we know this from history and it's just there. Every day you see...you see what can be holding you back, but you have no choice with it; you just have to go with it"*. (FG1).

Most of the participants also delved into their perception of the influence of history, including the slave trade, as playing a role in their view about not challenging unpleasant situations in their mental health experiences with services. It was expressed that the stories of the experiences of deprivation during the slave trade era was impacting on the behavior of the clients having 'no choice' in their interactions with the services. An example of this view is included in that Jane's statement in which she expressed also that there was a need for the clients to 'make a change for this generation':

> *"History, like our ancestors.... our parents.... our grand....you know, going all the way back through our life. You know, black people know...like...your parents tell, your parents tell you, their parents told them, their parents told them and so on. So, we know, it's not hidden. It's passed down through traditions, it's for us to try and make a difference and try and make a change for this generation. Well, they told you about the slave owners and being beaten when you didn't follow the rules and about torture and about being chained. You know, they told you about being deprived of food, being deprived of water and about taking the crops, taking the minerals, you...you just know about all these things. It is something that's not a secret and even today you see a lot of documentaries and so on, highlighting what has happened in the past and what has happened to various people. We have the odd few who have had the strength to break down barriers and that are*

> *who we have to thank for our strength today I suppose. If it weren't for them, we may be in a worse position."* (Jane, FG1).

This expressed view regarding a feeling of having no option than to take or abide by instructions from the health professionals without question or challenge, as a result of perceived historical norms would suggest the reason for the observed externality in LOC from most of the participants.

Another example of this perception of externality in LOC as emanating from historical perspective was expressed by most participants from the ambit of the perception by older generations that the health professionals were not to be challenged due to their higher educational status and knowledge. This perception has also been expressed in the parlance that the health professional was infallible, and their decisions should, therefore, not be challenged. The perception that this view has been passed as a cultural approach to the present generations by their parents and forebears has also been expressed as being responsible for the clients' view that expressing their views during their interactions with services was not only against the culture as handed down by their forebears, (as doing so would amount to challenging the skills, power and knowledge of the health professional); but was also not likely to make any difference to the service they received. This expression suggests that the externality in LOC is, therefore, based on the view that their opinions would not matter, and therefore not necessary. For example, in expressing this notion, Alison referred to what she described as the behaviour of the earlier generations whom she defined as being 'passive', as it was not within their cultural practice to challenge the decision of health care professionals, the feeling that the latter were 'always right' and that 'you don't challenge it':

> *"...Yes. Because at the end of the day a lot of people, especially our parents' and grandparents' generations were passive. They wouldn't have dared to challenge doctor's decision. At the end of the day, they knew that the doctor*

*is always right, and it has come down to my generation as well that unless you are in the medical profession, you don't challenge it; you just go along with it. At the end of the day who are you to challenge it if you don't' know anything different?" (*Alison, 1-1)

3.5. Summary –Theme 3

This superordinate theme and the corresponding subtopics have demonstrated that there exists an influence of culture on the LOC of the participants in this study in their experiences with services. It includes the importance they place on identity, family and their view regarding how the services perceive their culture as paramount factors that impact their perception of control in mental health settings and in their experiences with services. They also highlight the significance of culture in the formulation and maintenance of their identity; the significance of family in their culture, and their view regarding how the services perceive their culture as the subtopics. They view principally the absence of positive consideration of their culture by professionals as having led to their experience of inequality in treatment and care with services and their externality in LOC.

Most of the participants expressed a lack of control due to services ignoring their culture, the role culture plays on their sense of identity, the role of their family members and friends in their mental health challenges. They also expressed the view that the services did not only ignore their culture but also had an inferior view of the culture of the A & C clients. They also attribute the poor perception of their culture by services to the historical factors, the socio-economic issues as well as their own historical perspective, including parental and older generation's view that A & C clients should not challenge or question the authority of the health professionals.

These perspectives seem to have contributed to the externality in LOC of most of the participants within the mental health context. This theme has also highlighted the way in which most of the participants in this study attributed their perception of externality in their mental health LOC to issues that have impacted their mental health experiences, including culture and power. It also includes the participants' perception that they have no power to influence decisions made by services regarding their mental health due to the notion that they had inferior cultural, educational and socio-economic status as clients in comparison to those of the healthcare professionals from the mainstream population, particularly the psychiatrists. The latter are also viewed to have this notion of inferiority of the Black people's cultural, socio, educational and economic status, which, in turn, are considered by the participants as explanatory for the way the psychiatrists treat the Black clients by ignoring their culture and exercise power over them, thereby leading to externality in LOC in the clients.

The participants also attribute the cause of this perception of a lack of consideration for their culture by the psychiatrists as well as the clients' view of lack of control to historical and generational normative factors. This include the role of the slave trade and its perceived impact on the perception of low cultural status from the perspective of the psychiatrist and the normalised behaviour of not rocking the boat or drawing attention to oneself from the perspective of the clients. These suggest that these combinations of factors are viewed as leading to externality in the LOC of the participants.

4| Experiences of Care and Control

This superordinate section relates to participants' notion of experience of care and control. This includes their experiences at various stages- referral, assessment, treatment, and care. They have been subdivided into coercive practices, lack of consistent care, 'earning' discharge, and the perception that their personal needs were not being met.

4.1. Coercive Practices

Under this subtheme, most participants described their view of experiencing a loss of control over their lives from a perception of being forced into hospital admission. The externality in LOC were also contained in their hospital experiences, including the expressed perceived need to adjust or modify their behaviours and taking certain actions to please the professionals in order to receive needed attention, as well as into complying with the health professionals' directives against their own will.

An example of this perception of externality expressed in several description of feelings of a loss of power and authority in the experiences of admission, is contained in a description by Brian that his opinion was not considered in the entire process and decisions made regarding his hospitalisation were 'all done over my head':

> *"So, in my experience of my admission to hospital was that I had no power, I had no authority and it was all done for and all done over my head"*. (FG1).

Admission experiences were also expressed in the context of being without freedom. An example of this is indicated in admission being referred to by one of the participants as 'being locked up':

> *"I was not used to being locked up……. I was told I couldn't go home and I had to wait….. I didn't like that. I didn't like that at all, being locked up…I didn't like that at all"* (Bianca, 1-1).

In addition to the perception that they were not involved in decision making in the admission process, most participants also expressed that they felt that their experience in hospital was characterised by being pressured into taking medication. For example, Alan described his experiences of being physically forced to take medication as follows:

> *"…uuh it was a terrible place to be you know, the décor, the environment, it's so nasty. I wouldn't take medication, I was held down and given the injection, you know umm…. because you know at the time, I didn't think there was anything wrong with me so in the end it took about…a good 10 of them to hold me down. Not that I was fighting you know, I think they were just scared you know but I wasn't going to fight with them because I didn't see the point but in the end they called the security because at the time they wanted to hold me down to take the medication but ummm….".*(1-1).

Another example of this perception was expressed in a similar experience described by Brian, who indicated that he felt that he was subjected to 'punishment' for refusal to take medication:

> *"…. say for instance when I was in the hospital I was held down, I was held down now how many times? Now…….one……oh man, when they held me down, they held me down and they gave, me an injection in my backside man yeah…and then they put me in to an isolation room you know? There was a room you know that there was nothing in there, just a mat you know, and I thought "what the hell did they put me in here for?" But I was just playing it cool and I just laid down and that wasn't very*

good, that wasn't good. There was no need for that you know, I couldn't understand why, and it was almost like...like.... I have to have this medication you know...and if I don't you know....If it doesn't, I was going to be punished. So, I felt that, I refused to take the injection and that happened about 4 times and every time I'd end up in this room on my own you know?" (FG1).

The reaction of feeling of helplessness to being treated against their will was described by another participant, who expressed feeling having 'no will', feeling 'nothing' and feeling a sense of helplessness, and resigning to 'just take whatever they give you':

".......I was treated against my will upon admission to the mental health hospital.....having been treated against my own will....you have no will when you're in such a depressive state. You have no will...your will is gone...it's...it's.....you go along with whatever they give you because you have no will. There is no life, there is no enthusiasm, there is nothing, you are nothing, you feel nothing, you are nothing and you are really suicidal. That's the end of your life, you don't have any will, you don't want to live, that's it; you've had enough of this life. So, to be treated against your will, you have no will so you just take whatever they give you" (FG1).

This thought of resignation was also expressed by Carla who expressed a feeling of being 'brainwashed' in hospital, following rules and doing what one is told, not asking why and 'it's the rules':

"Oh right, well I dunno well I suppose they tell you to do things every day and sort of brain wash you type thing you know. Oh just, I dunno you just do things that you have been told isn't it. You do what you're told. You don't ask why sometimes with certain things, it's the rules so it's the rules" (FG2).

Many participants also expressed a variety of reactions to their perception of being subject to pressure to take medication during their hospital stay, which may have also contributed to their externality perception of LOC. The responses were characterised by a combination of different emotions, including refusal, pretence and acquiescence. In this vein Jane cited a scenario:

> *"...well I'd just say that I don't want to take it and they'd say that I had to take it. It wasn't literally a tantrum about it, it was just alright then I'll take it. Sometimes I wouldn't take it and pretend to take it and end up taking it. It didn't always happen that way."*

This perceived need for modification of behavior as a result of LOC externality perception was also expressed by Melanie in relation to the need to adhere to medication regime prescribed by the professionals, as she felt that doing otherwise could have resulted in detrimental consequences for her, including the likelihood of the refusal being placed on the patient's record, and this being consequently being viewed as 'noncompliance' and being seen as a non-cooperative patient, and which she described as being capable of being 'damaging':

> *"Well for example, medication. You are prescribed medication and if you...if you are having any problems with that medication and you decide not to take it, it's deemed as non-compliant. Non-compliant goes on your record and noncompliance is seen as you are not co-operating with the professional and that can be damaging for you."* (FG2)

The perceived coercion articulated by the majority of the participants, including the use of medication and the provisions of the Mental Health Act to continue detention due to non-compliance, which was indicated to have impacted on their externality in LOC, was also included in the recount of their hospital experiences in seeking and receiving support. It was expressed that being able to see the doctor by request or being allowed to go on day leave could only be achieved by adhering to conditions that were placed on them by the professionals. An example of this perception was indicated in Dennis' experience in which the word 'IF' was emphasised to illustrate the conditionality placed on requests by the clients:

> *"...you'll be allowed out IF you take extra medication, IF you take this first or IF you wait to see the doctor first" and there's no intention of the doctor coming along. The doctor mightn't even be around that day or whatever, or "you have to wait and see the doctor before you go out, we'll let you go out, you just have to wait and see the doctor" and they're waiting there all day. ..."* (FG1).

This perception was also expressed by Jane to the effect that it was necessary for the clients to use their 'skills' in order to negotiate their welfare:

> *".well...whilst your, whilst your under mental health, whilst your under the mental health team you do lack authority because as I said you have to comply, you have to comply with what is being placed in front of you. You have to .... use all of your skills that you have learned over the years to self-help because no one is going to help you apart from yourself". (*FG1).

Alan used a similar expression in describing his experience regarding decisions being made on his behalf without being asked, his response to that and his way of stating his opinion without challenging decisions made for him in order to manage his situation:

> *"...decisions were made for me and the only way I could influence them is by....is by...well, basically agreeing to what had been said and then coming back and saying my opinion on what that decision was. So, I did learn to.... I didn't really challenge any decisions because that wouldn't have helped the situation I don't feel. I was*

> *better off trying it, coming back and saying why I agreed with it or disagreed with it".* (FG1).

Many participants also expressed being coerced into reacting positively to the perceived power and control exerted by the health care professionals. For example, Jane commented that although she did not feel that the health care professional was right by saying that she needed medication, she eventually complied with the medication regime because:

> *"I didn't want to worry myself about anything too seriously wrong with me".* (FG1).

Brian contributed to this perception in one of the focus group settings in describing his response to this perception expressed by other participants that they needed to modify their behaviour to suit the exercise of power by the professionals:

> *".. Because it didn't make sense to prolong your agony or prolong your pain. I mean not everybody thinks like me of course because everybody's different but that is -my belief and that is what got me through. But if you don't have that inbuilt in you or have that support network that you've grown up to build up in you then of course everybody will react differently but that's what got me through".* (FG1).

Many participants also expressed that they found it difficult to express their opinion regarding their treatment experience, as they were reluctant to do so for fear of negative consequences. This was highlighted by Alan:

> *"....I find that my treatment...I try and be cool, I try and be calculated in terms of trying to express myself in an intelligent way and try to find out what they are trying to get at and then it depends on how they behave towards me. I have found in the mental health services, they don't like people to be articulate. They don't like people to*

express themselves. These are the people we are dealing with" (Alan, 1-1).

This statement by Alan including trying 'to be calculated' also indicates exercising internality in LOC in his interactions with services, suggesting that he was trying to exercise control over what he considered a negative condition. This perception was also explained in the context of controlling one's emotion in order to avoid creating a wrong impression:

> *"Well the only power and control that I would say I had was that I had to think, I had to think er... about my actions more so in depth because of who I was speaking to. So, I would say at time my power, my control was over my own emotions in order not to show signs of any behaviour which could be perceived wrong".* (Alan, 1-1).

Another example of this perception was expressed by Carla, who used the word 'punish' in describing the need to be calm and diplomatic in dealing with services:

> *".. Well unless, unless you can speak up for yourself and do it in a very diplomatic way and calm, I was calm; you will be sectioned, and you will be in trouble or reprehended or what do you call it? Apprehended. Yeah, yeah, they will punish you basically"* (FG2).

The perception of forced compliance to take medication and perceived fear that something might be seriously wrong if they did not take the medication was also expressed in terms of aftermath of feeling a continued sense of lack of control over their lives by many participants. This was expressed by a feeling of being tied to the mental health system due to the need expressed by the services for the participants to take medication. For example, Dwayne described this as a 'system ', and within which someone was being 'stuck' and unable to come out of as follows:

> *"That's what troubles us in the mental health system, if it wasn't for the medication, some of us wouldn't in the*

> *system. It's the medication that keeps us in there, that power and control; I call it artificial straight jacket. That's the system, no matter how you try to get out, how you try to go a different way. The mental health community, the system, you can't go there because you've got to go back for the medication next week, you've got to go back in, so you're stuck within the system because of the medication".* (1-1).

He expressed further that this experience with medication and compliance impacted on them as individuals, including a perception of being kept 'under the system':

> *"…but we are under spiritual strait jackets and the medication that they give us is part of that. This keeps you under the system, no control, no power, you lose your identity so you're a different person completely." (*Dwayne, 1-1)

The perceived lack of control was also expressed in the context of experience of fear on arriving at hospitals following admissions via coercive pathways. Some of the expressions include a feeling of fear and personal insecurity on admission. This led to sleepless nights for some. An example of this was contained in a statement by Alison, who seems to indicate that she still recalls her experience of being 'frightened to death', even after many years of being discharged. This seems to suggest that recalling these negative experiences may have impacted on externality in LOC:

> *"I couldn't sleep, I was always scared; frightened to death ummm".* (1-1).

These perceptions of feeling unsafe and coerced, (externality in LOC), were also expressed by statements which referred to the hospital as *"an awful place to be*"; "scary"; and a feeling of "being locked up".

Another example in this respect was also expressed in the context of perceived helplessness as described from an admission experience by Patricia as follows:

> *"...it was scary looking outside, it was awful. I couldn't get to sleep, I couldn't do anything. I had to wait till the morning before I could do anything and then you go to sleep. You see the carers, they don't sit with you well they said that they will sit with you until you fall asleep, but I didn't get there. I didn't get that care while I was there. So...I didn't hate anybody, but it was an awful place to be and to be mixing with people".* (FG1).

It was also found that although these experiences expressed by the participants occurred in some distant past, the perception of a lack of control due to their care experiences were also expressed in the context of perceived ongoing fear of readmission by most participants. In this respect, fear and a feeling of insecurity emerged as a common factor expressed by most participants years after they had been discharged from hospital. This includes fear of possible rehospitalisation, repeated trauma of being sectioned and reported panic attacks. The participants also expressed a need to be supported to deal with these fears they have experienced which contributed to their LOC externality, as support is also perceived as an important factor in their recovery. For example, Gerald expressed this feeling, including how the fear was still affecting his ability to feel safe:

> *"...so I can hardly walk the streets, I still think someone's going to lock me up or something umm....I panic a lot ummm....If I have to ...if I have to.. If I've got an appointment, I have to be on it all day because if I get up; I could go into a turmoil and forget that I've got to go somewhere. That never happened to me but that's what's happening, and I think it's a great pressure that's got to be dealt with and see how I get on"* (1-1).

Ryan also commented that he still experiences fear due to his experience of being admitted with the involvement of the police and his treatment in hospital:

> *"I would say the environment in trying to connect to all agents.... I then had panic attacks. Also, at home, I had little bits, some of arguments and all that....Whenever I think hard, they would use the sirens to disturb my mind, until now they are still following me wherever I go and that still causes me fear and panic attacks, to suppress me. And I have mentioned it to one authority, but they don't look into it"* (Ryan, 1-1).

This description which seems to suggest a feeling of suffering as a result of sirens disturbing the mind would connote a sense of lacking control over one's life (externality in LOC). This is also a sad scenario, given that the participant expressed that there has been no response from people of authority to requests to address the challenges.

Another example of this perception has also been taken from the experience of repeated admissions described by Adrian:

> *"That's what I would look at as coercion. They'd do that to me all the time, all the time. I'd get sectioned, be on the ward for a little while, they said I'm getting better, check whether I'm taking my medication or not, the doctor discharge me and I'd be at home. They turn around again and do the same thing. I might say something do them blah blah.... and we're just going round and round and round and round and in and out and in and out and out. I keep thinking it's going to change and it's not."* (FG1).

This perception of expected episodes of readmissions was also expressed from the context of the clients being surprised when the expected readmission does not occur. This is included in Adrian's statement in which he indicated that he could not believe that he was not readmitted again after so many repeated episodes:

"Over the last 13 years I haven't been in hospital, I just can't believe it, I can't believe it. Because from 1995 to 2003, most of that time I was in hospital. When I got out of hospital the last time I went back for 7 days and I got discharged, came out then and never looked back but I just used to keep thinking to myself they're going to turn around and just say well you have to come back in and I said to my mum "well, how am I expected to live like this?" (FG1).

This expression of almost suspecting that they could be readmitted at any time as indicated above is likely to lead to externality of the LOC of the individual, as a result of the perception uncertainty, and that they have no control over what might occur.

The perceived lack of control and consequent externality in LOC expressed by most participants attributable to the perceived experiences of coercive practices in their mental health experiences have been highlighted in this subtheme. It indicates that the participants' experiences of admission, assessment, hospitalisation were characterised by a feeling that control over decisions regarding these processes were out of their own hands, leading to fear of repeat of the experiences. This suggests further that a perpetuation of externality in LOC may have resulted, as the participants also expressed that they intend to avoid rehospitalisation due to this fear.

4.2. Lack of Consistent Care

Under this subtheme, participants responded to questions relating to their perception of control of their lives and their view of mental health care experiences. They were also asked to if they perceived that there was a link between the two issues and their culture. Most participants expressed inconsistency in the care they received, and this was construed as poor care, which they in turn expressed as having a bearing on their perception of control over their lives, as they felt that the inconsistency impacted on their ability to exert control on the processes of their care. It was also expressed that they perceived that they had no control over decisions regarding the care they received, which they, in turn, attributed to differences in culture. An example of this perception of experience of poor care is contained in Patricia's statement, including a feeling of being disheartened and sadness, and of a lack of fulfilment of 'obligation to take care':

> *"Well I actually ...I don't...I didn't....I didn't and don't feel looked after by the Mental Health Services. I feel that I was let down by an organisation that was set up to help me and many others and I find that quite disheartening and sad...Because it's an organisation that is a national health organisation and that is a public organisation which has been especially designed, built, developed for people that are unwell. So therefore, anything that you do within that organisation should be for the good of health and not for the detriment of health. So, if a person experiences anything that is negative which could have been avoided, that organisation is the wrong one you know; because at the end of the day that organisation didn't fulfil its obligation to take care".* (FG1).

Many participants also expressed a perception of experience of poor attitude by the health care staff in hospital wards, including a feeling of being ignored, which gave them a feeling of not being given control in their hospital experiences. An example of this perception is contained in Trish's description of the hospital being a 'horrible place to be', the nurses' not spending time with patients, ignoring them, and not having 'common courtesy'. He also describes this behaviour as being akin to 'not being paid proper money':

> *"I don't know, it's just that all I can say is that it's just a cold experience yeah, I didn't strike up any kind of relationship with any of the nurses in there, they feel like they're not being paid proper money. They told me that yeah (laughs), they spend a lot of their time in the....when I was on.....they spend a lot of the time in the office yeah and every time you*

want something you have to bang on the office door and they don't bloody look at you, you know, I found that really bloody annoying. You know just a simple thing like that, there wasn't even that common courtesy...I mean...It's a horrible place to be that's all I can tell you, I found it a horrible place to be and I couldn't wait to get out yeah and I don't know......" (FG2).

Perception of inadequacy of care was also expressed in the comments made in respect of mixing people with different types of illness together as well as an absence of talking or holding discussions with the patients by the health care staff. An example of this perception contained in Tim's statement includes the observation that the health care staff did not spend time with their patients, describes as 'no reasoning that went on, they haven't got the time...' and perceived mixing people with different diagnosis 'who are alcoholics and drug addicts' in the same environment:

".... there was no reasoning that went on either, there was no reasoning that went on. They haven't got the time for it, I don't know if they're getting paid for it. I don't know what's going on, but the atmosphere is terrible in hospital they really need to spend some money and look at giving people some kind of therapy, at least try to reach them in some kind of way, find out where they are you know. Also, you are in there with people who are alcoholics you know and drug addicts, nothing against them but I don't know if that's the ideal place for the two to meet. People with mental health problems...not people with mental health problems people with drug problems yeah....so it's a complex situation but you know.... It's very difficult, some people just don't look after their self. There's no real love in hospital.... there's no real love man". (FG2).

The perceived attitude of the hospital staff was also highlighted by Bryony in her statement, indicating the need to have a strategy to overcome' whilst in hospital, and being a 'target' and a 'victim'

> *"In terms of the care that I've had to be honest, I've been detained in mental health institutes; in the infirmary and I've learned that if you don't have a strategy to overcome what is in front of you then you're always going to be hit with Cupid's arrow. It could be a manager on the ward; it could be a patient on the ward who's out for your love life; to wreck your life, to whatever. It could be the chef in the kitchen. Someone there has just had a bad day and sees that you're a target and if you become a target, you will be a target and if you become a victim, you will be a victim".* (FG2).

The perception of poor care was also attributed by many participants to have emanated from perceived confusion by the healthcare professionals regarding having enough or adequate knowledge of the participants. Many of the participants expressed that this inadequacy of information has led to inconsistency in the care they received. An example of this perception was included in Jane's statement:

> *"...... they don't know what they're doing sometimes. One doctor will treat you one way and the next team will treat you a different way. You don't know who's who or what's going on, there's just sheer confusion".* (FG1).

The participant added that this confusion makes care problematic, adding:

> *"... if you are confused about someone you won't be able to care for them"* (Jane, FG1)

Differences in response for similar requests by the health care personnel was also highlighted as impacting on the perception of poor and inconsistent care experience. Examples of this perception include Patricia recount of experience, in which care was described as 'patchy' and 'inconsistent':

"Erm...it depends It did depend on who saw me, and it did depend on their workload but I must say, I found their care a little bit patchy. It wasn't consistent. Some people are in it for the right reasons and some people just are not and you just have to navigate your way through the system as best you can, with who is presented to you. At the end of the day I didn't find it totally consistent. I would have liked it to be consistent but at the end of the day that doesn't happen" (Patricia, FG1).

A sense of Patricia's disappointment over this perception was also expressed by Alison, including a description of varying degrees of 'level of care':

"Like, I know that no two people are the same but your level of care should be reflected from person to person but that wasn't the case. Some doctors, some nurses, some OTs ....it...it was so varied that I don't think it was conducive to good health".(1-1).

Another example of the perception of poor and inconsistency of care is found in a description of an experience by Melanie of what she perceived as a poor response to her call for support when she suspected that she was going through a relapse, and a lack of prompt response to her GP' referral by the mental health services:

"I feel that I know that I'm going downhill because I have an insight into my own illness and I felt that I was becoming a bit high, manic and I went to my GP and I was to be referred back to the team. I was waiting for quite some time to wait to hear from the mental health team and they weren't getting in contact with me and by then I was slowly getting worse and worse and worse so I had to go to Re-think which is the advocacy service and they wrote to the team and asked for an emergency appointment for me. I wasn't being seen quickly enough. There I wasn't being treated properly". (FG2).

This narration illustrates that LOC externality may be experienced when the client feels that they are unable to express their opinion about their health with the expectation that a prompt response will be received from professionals. The perceived poor care was also expressed by Jane, who highlighted her experience with the home treatment team (mental health teams who provide support at client's residences), as an example of a lack of consistency and joining up of information, constant change of staff which impeded relationship building, and staff prejudging her:

> *"Well they need to pass on information to one another properly, just pass on information between themselves; from one team to another. If I am going from hospital on a ward and then the home community team are coming to me, the home community team need to know what's being going on in hospital for me, who I am; what's been going on for me and they need to have the same person come to visit me. I found when I had the home community team come to visit me it was different people every day and so I couldn't build up a proper bond or relationship and to be honest with you, some of the nurses I didn't particularly like, you know and it was different nurses that were coming to my house every day".* (FG1).

The perception of poor care experience expressed by most of the participants in relation to their perceived loss of control were also described from their perception that the experience of care was linked to perceived cultural differences between the participants and the health care professionals. In this vein, most participants expressed experiences of differences in approaches and treatment by the health care professionals due to their cultural difference. In buttressing this perception many of the participants cited difference in response to their requests in comparison to the responses that their white fellow clients received. For example, Patricia stated that she perceived that the standard of care she received was low 'because I'm black' as follows:

> *"Well the care....the care I received wasn't' to the highest standard because I'm black"*. (FG1).

This expressed link between cultural differences and differences in care experiences was also illustrated in an example by Alison, including the perception that patients were treated 'according to the colour of their skin':

> *"I remember sometimes when I was on the ward; some of the staff used to treat people different according to the colour of their skin you know? If you were a white person they might, not necessarily be more hostile to you but if you asked for something there's more chance you'll get it before the black person will get it because it's something like a prejudice inside them"* (1-1).

Alison also attributed her perceived poor care experience to being attended to by a white professional, whom she perceived was not 'in tune' with her life experience due to cultural differences:

> *"Well put it this way, I was always faced by Caucasian white professionals so I suppose my culture played a role; in that I didn't feel that they were in tune to my life and what I was going through because how could they be?"* (Alison, 1-1).

Noella also expressed the perceived difference and inconsistency in treatment experience on account of cultural differences by citing an example of when she shared her experience with other clients who were White, stating that she believed that a comparative 'terrible time' between her experiences and those of white clients would indicate that there is a difference in levels of experience. This indicates that Noella was of the view that a white client's experience of poor service will be comparatively lower than her own experience of poor service as an A & C client, as she perceived that her own service experience would be worse than those of her white counterparts:

> *"Because there are many people....I know that there are white people that Caucasian white people will say that erm....they had a terrible time but once again; that's their interpretation. My terrible time and your terrible time, once we get talking are two very different terrible times. SO, until we come together and discuss this openly, you know some people what they call terrible I call like "oh that wasn't too bad compared to what I went through". They can't understand that you know, and it is all about. It is all about the level of care not being consistent".* (1-1).

This sentiment was also illustrated by Carla, in comparing her experience with her white counterpart, indicating that they reported to her that they were able to receive a higher level of support from her psychiatrist than she did:

> *"My level of support was very weak, very poor erm...I felt at the time I needed more support and I asked for more support and it wasn't given to me. I know white people under the same doctor, and they said to me when they asked for it, they got it"* (FG2).

Patricia also described a similar experience of what she considered as partiality in response to her *request by a psychiatrist, due to what she perceived as a difference in cultural background.* She also expressed disappointment at the differences in the experiences of other clients with the same psychiatrist in comparison to her own experience*:*

> *"Like, my psychiatrist he didn't provide me with the adequate support that I would have liked but speaking to people who were under the same psychiatrist at the time; they have said that umm.... of another back ground...they have said "oh he was always fantastic to me, he was great to me". I.....I couldn't quite work it out. I know that people are different to different people but at the same time you're not supposed to be a friend to people, you're supposed to*

be a doctor. He's in a position of quite high authority with medications and with your life as it were in his hands and I do feel that perhaps he had a personal thing. I couldn't quite put my finger on it at the time but in hindsight I was right". (FG1).

In expressing their experience of differences care, Patricia highlighted differences in response to personal care needs as an example of perceived differences in treatment due to cultural differences:

> *"In terms of white people on the ward, they might have sore legs or things like that, and they make sure that have creams things like that for them and whatever. You know, they just make sure they, they're looked after and then they have people of colour or whatever and they're not looked after; they're just not looked after. There's no cream….no, no, no, no, no they haven't got any"* (FG1).

In a similar vein Bryony described feeling treated differently from people of other cultures, as she received different types of care due to her physical appearance as a mixed-race patient, although she self-described herself as a Caribbean. She stated that the difference in treatment approaches was influenced by the health professional and the prevailing circumstance at the time of treatment:

> *"…because I am mixed race there have been times that I have been treated like a white person and times I have been treated like a black person….by the way that they treat me, the questions they ask me, ermm….the medications they try to put me on, the way they speak to me, the diagnosis they try to give you. Just different things"* (FG2).

> She *added:*
> *"It's bizarre because when I'm treated as a white person I'm treated as ah….somebody with a moderate to mild depression …erm…coherent, you know…capable…whatever.*

> *But them when I'm treated like a black person I'm treated as quite unstable, quite unwell, you know...things like that. It's.... it's bizarre and it's not me in my illness, it's the way I perceive it. It's the way it's coming at me"* (Bryony, FG2)

These statements highlight a link to the external notions of identity. As discussed in earlier chapters in this thesis, the grouping of individuals according to appearances and physical features plays a role in discrimination and stereotypes. This also raises another gap in research into the experiences of people of mixed ethnic backgrounds, their sense of identity, their mental health and the responses of the services to them.

A similar issue was also contained in a response by Alan who expressed his observation that there is a difference in the way Black people are approached by the professionals in comparison to their white counterparts in the hospital wards:

> *"It's the way they speak to the black people, it's very abrupt, rude, disrespectful and I've seen how they speak to the white people. They are very polite and gentle and sort of they empathise with them and understand them or they .... if they don't understand them, they try to. They're not as cautious around white people, they're more cautious or seem to think they are going to be attacked or something by a black person".* (1-1).

Another example of this perception was by Alan in which he added by describing a characteristic of Black people being loud, singing, and dancing in ward settings, which may be construed as indication of mental illness, as a result of a lower level of understanding of their culture:

> *"...to be honest, some of us may be a little bit loud. But it's our culture that we're loud, we speak loud, or we might sing or dance and it's not because we're ill, it's our culture. Some of us are actually happy, and dancing and we get "Go to your room, get more medication, go for an*

> *injection, you need more medication" things like that"* (Alan, 1-1).

This perception of low awareness of culture by health professionals was also attributed to differences in the way the professionals treat clients from the A & C groups in comparison to people from other cultures. An example of this perception is contained in Adrian's experience of ward visits (as a trained client peer supporter), in which he also described his perception of the differences in behaviour on account of culture, the exercise of power by the health care professionals in response to their misunderstanding of this, as well as the consequent difference in treatment of patients from the Black populations in comparison to those from the mainstream population within similar contexts:

> *"The power is where they'll tell them, if they're a bit boisterous or they might be singing; they might actually be singing because they're happy. They'll tell them to "shut up! Go to your room! Stop making noise! You need more medication, you need to be calmed down." If they're knocking at the office door for a reason they'll be told "go away, you're a nuisance, come back later, we haven't got time now". Whatever, they haven't got time for them. That's black people. If it's a white person, I've seen it and I've heard it, "within two minutes, just stay there, we'll be out in two minutes". If they're knocking at the office door, if they're singing or whatever they'll say, "oh you're very happy". They will interact with them, they will engage with them "oh you're happy today, what are you singing, that's a lovely song". They might even join in and sing with them"* (FG1).

The foregoing has highlighted the perceptions and the accompanying statements and scenarios contained in the experiences of the participants which were cited as factors that combined to contribute to their perception of externality in LOC. This is due to the perception expressed that their care were not up to standard due to the perceived differences in their culture, the exercise of power by the professionals based on their culture and the perceived differences in levels of support they received from their psychiatrists in comparison to those received by their white counterparts for the same need combined to make them feel that the control of their mental health experiences were not in their own hands but in the hands of people outside of themselves.

4.3. 'Earning' Discharge

In this subtheme under perception of experiences of care and control, participants expressed further their perception of a lack of control of their circumstances whilst in hospital. The main notion expressed by most participants related to a perception that they had no control over decisions regarding their discharge from hospitals, which necessitated that they had to perform certain acts or behave in certain manners in order to be discharged from hospitals. One example of this perception is contained in Bianca's description of a feeling that their actions were controlled by services professionals, and the need to 'calm down' and 'conforming':

> *"They have control over your actions and behaviour because at the end of the day you want to be discharged, so if you want to be discharged there is only one way to get discharged. You cannot get discharged by being unreasonable or erratic or....even though you may feel that you want to be this way. You can't get discharged behaving in this manner. Most people learn that the hard way but that is a fact. Until you start to calm down and start erm...I don't know....conforming, this is the only way you're going to get discharged so if more people had that viewpoint then perhaps we wouldn't have so many people in treatment". (1-1).*

Modification of behaviour was also expressed in this perception of lack of control and externality in LOC. For example, Alan illustrated the need to 'get better in order to come out' and 'being as good as you can'. This suggests that one must jettison one's rights to control one's life in order to be discharged:

> *"I was in there for 6 months.... I .I couldn't take it where I was but I had to get better in order to come out. That means just sitting a lot and............and being as good as you can"*. (1-1).

This perception of relinquishing one's control, and adopt a state of externality in LOC in order to 'earn' discharge was also expressed as the need to be of 'good behaviour' by Mary:

> *"put it this way I um....I didn't like the hospital and ...I wanted to just do good behaviour as much as I could to come out of there. Um...there were no thoughts of me....um....things were quite bad so..."* (1-1).

In another example in highlighting this perception along with the role of perceived power of the health professional in promoting externality in the clients, Alison articulated that the ability of the clients to 'go along with' expectations of the health professional will likely lead to positive results for their request for discharge. She also expressed the fear of the consequences of not complying which may in turn impact negatively on what she described as being 'released':

> *"You know, when you go and see the psychiatrist and they say, "how are you feeling today" and so on and so forth and you need to explain and some days you're able and some days you're not. That would mean "oh, you need your medication increased". So.....but....it's not that, it's not that.....so you go along with it because you feel that you have to go along with it because it's been prescribed for you and you weren't forced to go along with it. You were given it though knowing that you basically had no choice. Well, you took it like I said....well you could just not take it but like I said, it would just be increased and if*

> *you're of the mind-set that you don't want it increased you just take it. You just take it so you can be released"* (1-1).

This subtheme has highlighted the externality in LOC of most participants being promoted by their perception of a lack of control in decisions regarding their discharge from hospital by the mental health services. This include the perception that they had to 'earn discharge' by modifying their behaviour to suit the expectations of the professionals. The act of relinquishing one's control and handing it to external bodies is a feature of externality in LOC. Participants also expressed a feeling of seeking to be 'released' from hospital, indicating a perceived need for freedom from incarceration, as opposed to being supported in their mental health experiences.

4.4. Personal Needs Not Being Met

Under this subtheme of perception of care and control, most of the participants expressed their perception of a lack of control in their experience of services from the perceived unmet personal needs. This includes the perception by most participants that their voices were not being heard, as they were not being listened to, the perception that they had to 'fight' to receive care, and a perceived lack of personal support after discharge from hospital, which in turn leads to externality in their LOC. An example of the feeling of not being listened to by health care professionals was expressed by Jane, who expressed a feeling of being 'tokenistic', and a desire not to be listened to and not treated as a 'tick box' exercise:

> *"...sometimes, it does depend on what the situation is but sometimes my ....I feel, I feel tokenistic and....I ....I tried to highlight that. I don't really want to be tokenistic, I want to be listened to, I want to be heard, I want to be understood and I want what I say to be taken seriously not to be a tick box exercise as is and has been the case".* (FG1).

Another example of the perceived lack of voice is contained in a description by one participant who explained her ward visit observation in highlighting that members of the community are not being supported with their skin care needs:

> *"I actually visit the wards as a volunteer and there are people on those wards that their care needs are not being met. When I talk about care, I mean their personal care. Some people need creams for their skin because they have dry skin and ok some white people do but a lot of black people have skin problems, dry skin and things like that and there's none of that care and some of the ladies need special creams for their hair and special shampoo, not just every day shampoo but special shampoo that you can buy. They haven't got that supplied to them either and you know it's just care like that"* (FG1).

Another example in this respect relates to the perception that clients were not listened to and their views were ignored, as expressed by Leonie, who objected to the act of the professionals focusing on medication or intervening by isolation only in response to some perceived expression of psychosis by the clients:

> *"A lot of these people who are on the ward, yes they may be ill and they may be in a psychosis but I still feel that behind their psychosis and behind that psychotic episode there's a voice and there's a message and they're not listening to that, or they're listening to what they're coming out with and then they're saying "oh, more medication" or "go to your room", whatever else, they're not listening to exactly what's behind that voice. That's what I feel seriously"*. (Leonie, FG1).

This example indicates that a feeling of not being listened to on the understanding that someone was expressing some psychotic symptoms is likely to amount to ignoring issues that are likely important to the person at the time, thereby leading to externality. In addition, a decision to increase the medication or send the person to their room are likely to increase their externality in LOC, as they are likely to perceive that they have no control or are unable to receive support for the challenges they are going through.

Another example of this perception of externality includes the description made by Dwayne who expressed that he experienced a lack of access to what he needed, and having to 'battle' or fight to access support:

> *"Because I had to basically.......everything I have seen and want to achieve, I had to kind of fight for it. It wasn't' easily accessible to me. It wasn't easy. A lot of things that I have achieved there or tried to achieve there haven't been a walk in the park. You have to keep battling and battling and I don't think mental health organisation should require people to battle. I think it should be open, willing and .....more transparent in its actions".* (1-1).

This view also indicates that although this would suggest an attempt to take control of a situation within which one has no control, it also suggests that a feeling of not being able to exert enough pressure to achieve desired outcome may also lead to further extension of externality in LOC. This is due to the likelihood that the clients may start to feel that their effort is not likely to be rewarded, thereby leading further to externality in their LOC.

Participants also expressed lack of ongoing support for their recovery after discharge. This includes absence of support in community mental health settings. Brian described his experience with a social worker in which support was discontinued after two years, in spite of his expressing a desire to have ongoing support:

> *"So, I didn't stop seeing the social worker, all I said to the social worker is that I wanted to move into voluntary...you know, seek it out. So, he thought that I wanted to stop seeing him and that's not what I wanted; I wanted to share that experience with him of doing things but he didn't see that either. So, you see if I had a person, who*

could have shared my life a little bit longer; that would have helped". (FG1).

The expression of having one's support withdrawn in this example due to a misunderstanding of the intent and expressed need of the clients may have also led to the clients feeling a sense of externality in LOC, due to their perceived lack of control over the decision to discontinue support in their situation.

Participants also expressed a feeling of a lack of direction for control of their lives due to inadequacy or a lack of support. They also expressed the impact of this on their recovery. An example of this is contained in Alan's statement in which he expressed feeling a sense of loss of direction in his recovery:

> *"...... but you know it's like a step that I'm looking for...a step...a step... a step to recovery to stay there and let things roll for me. I don't know what directions to go. Yeah, I don't know what direction"* (1-1).

The externality in LOC in this example indicates that the client is likely to feel that they are not in control over their situation, as it is beyond their ability to achieve desired change through support.

Within the feeling of lacking control following their hospital experiences, many participants also expressed feeling that they perceived lack of knowledge or ability to commence improvement to wellbeing and control of their lives. Brian's statement illustrates this view that he was unable to see the possibility of a change for the betterment in his situation:

> *"As an individual .....to improve.........I can't say things to improve from what it is now ....., I can't say that. I have to work with a community organisation and if there' s something that you can change you can talk but I haven't reached those stages yet so..."* (FG1).

An expression of a lack of positive outlook for the future as indicated in this example is also linked to externality in LOC.

This perception of inadequacy of post discharge support was also expressed by many participants from the ambit of being able to relate positively in the community, the need to increase their communication skills and interactions with others. These are the areas of need for which many participants expressed is lacking for them after they have been discharged from hospitals. An example of this view is contained in Dwayne's statement in which he described his need in area of social skills and abilities, and which he expressed that the services were 'not so helpful' to provide long term support:

> *"You know in terms of if I needed help with a benefit they'd try to help with that or whether I needed help with a property they'd try to help with that and if I needed help with initially settling in to independent living they'd kind of help with that. Long term things with kind of long term help in developing yourself, developing my kind of social skills or social abilities .....those are the kind of areas that they've been not so helpful"*. (1-1).

As these expressions are made within the parlance of feeling that one is dependent on needs which are not forthcoming, it would suggest that externality in LOC is not necessarily limited to an ability to exert influence. It suggests that externality, as linked to a feeling of lack of control as expressed by many of the participants here, is also linked to a feeling that support is not forthcoming from where it is expected, thereby leading to a further sense of externality in one's LOC.

The perception of a lack of control and externality in LOC highlighted within this subtheme were also expressed by most participants within the context of unmet personal needs, particularly after their discharge from hospital.

4.5. Summary-Theme 4

This theme has described the issues that the participants have expressed as having had impact on their LOC from their experiences of care and control with services. It includes the expression of what has been indicated as coercive practices, absence of consistency in the care they received, the perception that they had to 'earn' discharge, and the experiences of their personal needs not being addressed by services. The experiences also seem to indicate some differences in the level of perception of control, as well as suggest a continuation of the perception of externality expressed by the participants within the contexts of admission processes and their hospitalisation experiences. This contrasts somewhat to the expressed initial perception by many participants that they had some level of control by being discharged, which indicated that they had some level of internality in LOC, as they were in control of their freedom in terms of being 'released' from hospital. It, thus, suggests that this internality status whilst discharged may now be tempered by a perception that they had to now 'fight' for care and post discharge support, which also indicates a response to externality in LOC.

5| Suggestions for Improving MHS Experience for African and Caribbean Clients

5.1. Introduction

In the final stages of the interviews conducted in both one-to-one and focus group settings, the participants were asked to express their opinions on what they perceived as the way forward in relation to what they had expressed as concerns during their experience with services. As the questions were asked with a view to soliciting their opinions on ways by which they felt that their concern regarding their expressed lack of control as well as differences in levels of control over their mental health experiences, this superordinate theme contains most participants' ideas in response to the question regarding how they perceive that the mental health services could improve their experiences as clients from the A & C community.

The subtopics identified within this include various suggestions made by the participants regarding staffing to include people from BME background, especially A & C people, to ensure that staffing are representative of the clientele including senior roles for A & C peoples; the need for healthcare professionals to show interest in the culture of the clients from the two populations; the need to listen to ideas of clients and their family members and include them in decision making; some suggestions relating to input by service users from A & C groups; and some suggestions regarding the involvement of members of the A & C communities, and suggestion relating to post discharge support.

5.2. Staffing By African and Caribbean, Including Senior Roles/Models

Within this subtheme, participants perceive that staffing should include more people from A & C populations. They also expressed that the mental health staff in senior positions should include people from the A & C community. They also expressed that these members of senior staff should act as role models that could impact positively on the experiences of the clients from the community. An example of this view is contained in Bryony's statement that there was a need to have Black people to be given senior roles in services as well as act as role models of support for Black clients:

> *"The only way we can make a difference is if there are more role models in the system and I mean role models that ARE in the system and able to be themselves. It would be nice if black people could be given the opportunity to have more senior roles with the view of ...shaping the top and helping the black service users along the way"* (FG2).

In describing her experience, Jane also insisted that such role models will be able to impact on the situation by not 'towing the line':

> *"...it would be nice if the.....the....if a lot of black people could go into the field of um.....ummm mental health and I don't mean go into the field just for financial gain. I mean with the respect of their colleagues and with the intention of looking after people of colour because we can have black people in the job but there's no point in having them in the job if they don't.....if they're just going to toe the line. I mean, what's the point? I mean don't get me wrong, there are Caucasian and white people in the post that are very warm and receptive but I wasn't fortunate to have them under my care, but I do know they're there".* (FG1).

These expressions seem to suggest that there is a need for people from the Black populations to be involved in shaping the services to suit the needs of the minority community members, due to the over representation of these populations. It also seems to indicate that most participants would prefer professionals from within the community to be employed and be empowered to challenge the observed current unsatisfactory condition they have expressed to have experienced. It is interesting to note that although there is a noticeable number of Black professionals in the mental health services; however, the concern appear to be expressed by the participants that these staff members are not in decision making and policy making positions and are, therefore, unable to address the mental health challenges of the A & C peoples in particular and BME mental health in general.

The idea expressed of 'not towing the line' also seems to suggest that the participants were illustrating 'toeing the line' in the parlance of taking actions that is different from the set out rules that they expressed as having been detriment to the issues such as recognition of cultural differences, involvement of family members, and other issues raised. This connotes the need for a bottom up approach whereby health professionals who are members of the A & C populations could support clients from the similar backgrounds by applying their knowledge and experience of their cultural needs.

The expressions above also indicate that there is a desire by the participants for people from within the two respective populations to be involved in managerial roles in order to be able to exert some form of influence in the services received by the service users from A & C groups.

This notion also seems to have emanated from the view that people from within the groups will be more aware of the needs of the communities, the importance of diet in their respective cultures as well as be able to identify with the challenges including the socio-economic issues facing the populations, their relationship to mental health challenges as well as their recovery journeys. In addition, it seems that the study participants' opinion regarding the need for professionals from the A & C groups to act as role models for clients are likely to be from the premise that it will act as increasing their LOC by encouraging them to aspire to adhere to health strategies towards recovery, as well as encourage them to aspire for higher achievement.

5.3. Non Black Professionals to Show Interest in the Culture of African and Caribbean Groups

Under this subtheme, most of the participants expressed that it was necessary for the health care professionals who are not from the Black population to show interest in the culture of the people they serve who are from the A & C background. Jane's statement illustrates this, in which she urged the professionals to increase their knowledge of the people including their background, skills, gifting and share with other professionals, in order to be able to support them better:

> *".. I think that the professionals should help the BME, as I said before is examine us, look at our talents, look at what we're gifted at, look at our background, look at our skills, check out our hobbies and share with each other...simple as that, share with each other"* (FG1).

This was also highlighted in Alison's opinion that the members of staff should spend some time in the community they serve in order to familiarise themselves with the culture of the people:

> *"Well I think they need to be in the community, they need to come out of the offices and the meetings and start engaging with people on the floor as it would be erm... That's the only way that you're going to know people is if you actually embrace them, engage, communicate, and reach out. You can't be sitting in a big office and expect to say, "oh I know about people" and you don't even talk to them on a daily basis or a weekly basis. You have to actually engage, mix erm....be a people person really in order for there to be any change"* (1-1).

This view was also expressed by Bianca, who expressed the need for the professionals to 'embrace' groups in order to learn about them, their life experiences, and avoid what she referred to as 'tokenistic':

> *"... if you're not willing to embrace that you can't learn about people, it would be impossible and even though someone may tell you "oh a particular group of people like to be treated this way" I still feel that you have to know if for yourself. It's all well and good for them saying...just for an example...."oh we have BME this and BME that" but BME this and BME that is not the answer. You know, what do YOU know? What do you know from life experience not what someone's told you and until you're willing to ...go out there ...I think as I said...as I mentioned earlier about Tokenistic... this is where the system is being let down? Nobody wants to go out there, everybody is willing to delegate"* (1-1).

Alison also stated that mixing with the community members will enable the professionals to gain more understanding of the health care needs and expectations of the people:

> *"That's where they would come into the community and engage and want to know. There are many communities within....within any given town in this country and in order to understand it you have to mix, you have to get involved, you have to understand. You have to be willing to take time out to do all this. You, you have to know how erm......you know...a particular people want to be treated. You have to understand the cultures, the beliefs, the processes that different groups of people go through"* (1-1).

This was also expressed by Brian who added that understanding of the attitudes and cultures of the people in the community can end the perception that the study population could be aggressive. He cited examples of the way some people may communicate with hand gestures, which may also be misconstrued as aggression:

> *".... a lot of mental health professionals are not understanding of cultures and their behaviours and their*

> *attitudes and their communication methods. So, interpretation is a lot of the time perceived by the Psychiatrist as aggressive and it's not aggressive, it's the way how that individual communicates, but it could be loud. It could be with their hands...it could be standing up you know. But that's how...that's how a particular group of people may wish to communicate with each other. It's all about interpretation..."* (FG1).

This statement seems to highlight the need for therapeutic communication (Bhui et al, 2013). In buttressing the point about the need to understand the behaviours of people as indicated by their cultures, Brian also cited an example that individuals within the A & C populations could be misunderstood when they experience upsetting situations or psychological challenges, which could lead to actions being taken that, may result in such individuals being sectioned or arrested:

> *".. I think that is why there are so many black people being picked up on sections and um..and if you notice that when they are picked up; once they have had a sleep or whatever they are....they are discharged back to the community because they were just upset or annoyed at that given time and then they are discharged but after seeing that it was just an episode. It wasn't just that they were you know; mentally mad it was just that they were upset about something that happened at home. It escalated to the street and then they're picked up without just cause"* (FG1).

Jane expressed that members of the profession also need to engage with the service users' culture to increase their understanding; she cited examples of understanding some culture-specific events could also lead to further understanding of the people they look after:

> *"Engage, engage with them, engage, mix erm, perhaps even have awareness you know; have awareness of*

> *particular events in particular cultures and then they could say "oh! I understand that now". Because you know we don't understand everything, we have to be open to learning and I think that's the only way that the trust...or any organisation really strengthens its membership and strengthens its appreciation of the society we're living in in general"* (FG1).

The perceived need for the professionals to seek to understand the cultures of the A & C groups was also expressed in the context of the need to be provided for the professionals to be provided training on the cultures of the people they serve in mental health services in order to understand how to meet their needs. An example of this view is contained in Mary's statement that professionals need to be provided 'specialised training' to enable them to understand the needs of the service users from the A & C populations:

> *"Well, they need to have some specialised training, I know that's a terrible thing but they do and know how to meet these people's cultural needs. They need to have specialised training and they need to hear and realise and understand what these people require"* (Mary, 1-1).

Part of Brian's statement in this regard also indicates that training could lead to a better appreciation of the cultures, history and needs of the service users from the A & C populations by the professionals and lead to better care:

> *"They could care for them by understanding their mental health, understanding their culture where they're from, their needs, their history. Things like that and listen to them, listen to what they need. That's very important"* (FG1).

The foregoing suggests that the participants' perspective on how the experiences of the A & C service users, as part of the BME groups could be improved if more people from the respective groups are involved in the care services. The understanding of the role of culture is also perceived to be necessary for better approaches as it will lead to a better understanding of the issues that are linked with the mental illness experiences of the service users from the A & C populations. These issues include an appreciation of the historical factors, socio-economic issues, and cultural attitudes to mental illness.

The participants also pronounced that it is important for the health professionals who are not from the BME backgrounds to embrace the idea of engaging more with service users from within the respective A & C populations in order to understand them better and to be able to consider their observations in their interventions with them. The issue about training of the professionals in cultures has also been highlighted and indicates that the services need to apply more funding into education about cultural diversity and the needs of specific cultures for more positive health outcomes.

5.4. Involving, Listening to Ideas of Clients, Family Members and Friends

As a follow up to the expressed concern by the participants regarding a lack of voice in their experiences with services, this subtheme contains the suggestion by the participants in this regard. It includes the recommendation that the health professionals should liaise and consult with clients and people that matter to them on issues regarding their care experience. It also includes the perceived need for friends and members of the extended family to be involved and encouraged to take part in the health care process. An example of this recommendation in relation to the services' approach is included in Dwayne's opinion that the professionals need to express compassion with their clients, and ask them how things could be improved for them:

> *"... all they need to do is sit down with that person and say "look, what do we need to do to make changes?" Sympathy and all things like that but they're not thinking of it like that they're thinking of medical because it's an NHS hospital"* (1-1).

This also includes the expression that the views of the clients regarding their experiences with services need to be sought by the professionals. Many participants also expressed surprise that their experience in hospital had not been shared prior to their participation in interview for this study expressing that they had not been asked to share their experience with mental health services by the professionals. For example, Alison stated that her experience with the one-to-one interview has led to a reflection on the fact that no one had asked her view of her experiences in hospital:

> *"I'm sitting here talking and no one has asked me all these questions".* (1-1).

Another example of this view is contained in Ryan's comment that the interview with him had led to him being 'woken up' to the realisation that no one had asked regarding 'what was it like' for him:

> *".., It's just been woken up in me that I haven't said much, I haven't said much from hospital to here and people haven't asked what was it like for you but there hasn't been an end because I'm still in it so....but it's just the treatment now, isn't it?"* (1-1).

These illustrations seem to suggest that a perception that the experiences of the clients from the A & C populations as minority groups have not been taken into account in the service provision, in spite of the fact that they are overrepresented in the services. It, therefore, highlights the importance of including their views in policies and service provision. Another example of the expressed need to involve family members is included in Noella's statement in which she indicated that family members make up the community, and the need for services to include involving families in what she recommended as 'breaking down barriers' and 'build bridges':

> *"...breaking down barriers, building bridges with the community and developing a community of people within the community and those communities of people are people*

> *with mental health problems. Not just them alone but their families and their friends should be there with them because some of the treatment and some of the care are in that family"* (1-1).

The expression of the need for the professionals to support members of the A & C population who want to support members of their family and friends who are mental health clients, also suggests the importance the participants ascribe to family members and their involvement in supporting individuals with mental health challenges. This view was also included in Adrian's statement that extended family system (which includes the involvement of cousins, aunties and other members of the family, in contrast to the nuclear family system), need to be recognised and taken into consideration by services:

> *"Black folks have got extended families. Auntie may want to help as well, and grandma may want to help as well. You know we've got to make it exciting for them to want to help us and get into the system, get into what we're talking about, get into issues around mental health services because they are your family"* (FG1).

By indicating the need for the involvement of extended family members such as 'grandma and auntie' to be encouraged in the care process by making it 'exciting' highlights the importance placed by the A & C service users to their families and their involvement in their mental health experiences. This also seems to contrast with the expressed notion of stigma impacting on the relationships within family members. It also suggests that the involvement of family members in visiting and being part of the decisions of their members with mental health challenges, including the extended family system by services may be a positive factor in increasing internality in the LOC of the clients from these populations. It also suggests that such consideration may lead to addressing stigma and attainment of more positive experiences and health outcomes.

Ryan also described in his statement the need to involve friends in the mental health experiences, by indicating that the initiative should also come from of clients. He also expressed that it would be less challenging by getting support from others:

> *"If you really can't talk to them about where you're coming from then it should be friends like, say "look, I want you to come with me to my meeting with my doctor, I've got my CPS meeting and they said I could bring a friend. Yeah bring a friend and they can stick up for you there so that will show the doctor that you've taken the initiative by bringing someone with you. If it's one thing I have learned is that you can't do it alone, you need someone else do to it, no one's an island"* (1-1).

Ryan's position here seems to suggest that the presence of a friend could not only boost their confidence in their interaction with the health professional. It also indicates that the presence of the friend who 'can stick up' for the client could reduce externality from the perceived lack of control over their relationship with the professional and increase the internality of the LOC of the clients. He also referred to the likely reaction of the Doctor observing that one had 'taken the initiative' may also have some positive impact on the LOC.

5.4. Post Discharge Support

As an offshoot of the expressed concerns by the participants regarding external control post discharge, this subtheme highlights the contributions of the participants to address these concerns. Participants expressed that the mental health services should provide support to the clients after they have been discharged. This has been expressed as a necessary step to avoid rehospitalisation. An example of this view is contained in Dennis' statement that there was a need to be further supporter with their medication and other issues in order to avoid them returning to what led to their illness in the first place:

> *"Well the only thing that can be done is...when a person is discharged...the only thing that can be done is for them to*

have...for them to have is better support, so that they don't slip back into whatever bought them there in the first place. That could be in many forms but whoever the person is that's got that is a loved one or somebody ....should be supporting that person ...to stop them....well for example not taking their medication. Keep an eye on your loved one" (FG1).

The statement b Brian highlights the need to consider the social background of the person before they became unwell in order to ensure that the after-discharge support is focused on ensuring that they did not return to the social pressures that might have led to their illness. Another example of the need to address social issue is contained in Alan's expression that after hospital support should also address isolation, for people who are by themselves. This includes citing an example whereby people are discharged into living alone in hostels and flats without considering the negative impact on loneliness:

"A lot of people don't have anybody. They are just sent back to their flats or sent back to a hostel and erm..that's the end of it you know. They are just discharged and put back out into the community without any support mechanisms in place". (1-1).

The foregoing indicates that, as loneliness and isolation may have contributed to mental illness in the first place, it is imperative that discharge plans should include strategies to ensure that the client is not returned to isolation or lonely states that may exacerbate their illness or lead to relapse.

In further reference to post discharge support many participants also expressed the need for the services to encourage peer support amongst their clients. Patrick's statement illustrates this view of having someone who can support and guide them, as important for stopping what he referred to as 'revolving door':

> *"I feel that's the only way to stop revolving door, to have somebody; doesn't matter who...just have that peer support erm...project worker...co-ordinator...somebody... who is interested in that individual and will sort of guide them through until they're strong enough to take care of themselves"* (FG1).

The support post discharge has also been expressed from the context of building people's skills and by providing them the opportunity to access training to meet their needs. Jane's statement in this regard suggested that support for training and building what she referred to as 'life skills' and 'social skills' which they might have lost due to long hospitalisation is important after discharge:

> *"Well they could offer better therapist and training and workshops and um different people have different needs. You know, life skills....some people don't know how to shop or budget, things like that. Or they have lost those skills and social skills".* (FG1)

Participants also frequently commented on the need for places where clients could go to receive support in the community. This includes drop in centres, as expressed by Dwayne:

> *"I recommend that there should be more mental health drop in centres or centres for people with issues and things like that and where they can get support and so there can be early intervention if need be"* (1-1).

While highlighting the need to address loneliness, Jane also expressed the need for places in the community where clients could be engaged in activities and be supported with advice and companionship in order to aid their recovery after their hospital experience:

> *"Well if there could be a centre or a home or a meeting place and invite people or have an open day or something. Invite people along and let them know what's going on and what it entails and see who's interested and let it be open*

to both males and females. The centre could offer advice, point them in the right direction. You know, if it's addiction, if it's mental health, you know if it's both. Offer them support, advice, companionship, a place to come and be and feel part of society..... and not be so isolated. A lot of them might hang out together but deep down inside are very lonely". (FG1).

In expressing regret that a day hospital which supported him in the past has been closed, Brian expressed that getting early support can prevent relapse, and that there should be centres in the community to provide such support:

"There used to be a day hospital there and they've shut down and even I attended that at one time and I found it very helpful. That actually prevented me from going back on the ward, readmitted, that day hospital did...Sometimes if the person is helped early....the majority of the time if a person is helped early, it can stop them from getting any worse and this is where the community could come in to put all these things in place" (FG1).

Participants also expressed the need for peer support in the community support centres for mental health clients in order to support each other. Carla suggested that having 'buddy system' could be helpful to identify any relapses and support each other:

"But if they could build up a buddy system or peer system support..something. A...a network erm... where they can at least go once a week even. Just so someone can keep an eye on and say that he or she is doing well or "oh dear, I think something may be happening with that person" and nip it early. All we're trying to do is nip things early because we know we can't cure but we can catch things early and stop them escalating into a worse situation. Buddy system of peer support" (FG2).

Participants also expressed the need for the professionals to get to know their clients by spending time interacting with them, in order to support them: Alison expressed the benefit of this in enabling them to be able to find out and understand their needs better by spending time with them:

> *"By interacting more with them....By going through their files if they're allowed and things like that and emmm ....yes the best way is interacting more with them and asking them their needs and things like that. Try spending time with them".* (1-1).

The foregoing indicate that the expression of post discharge support from the participants encompass the need for more interactions with the clients in order to understand their needs, the need to ascertain the social conditions of the clients before they became unwell and to address such conditions with a view to ensuring that a repeat of such impact does not occur. It also includes the need to encourage peer support and buddy system amongst the clients, as well as to empower them by training them on the social skills that they may have lost due to their hospital experiences. Participants also indicated that isolation should be addressed in order to tackle relapse. This has also been expressed in the form of a need to have dropped in centres where people with experience of mental illness can socialise and have a sense of belonging, in addition to taking part in activities within places where members of the A & C populations can support them and thereby promoting social inclusion.

5.5. Community Approaches- What the Community Members Must Do To Improve Mental Health for Their Members

Participants also expressed the need for members of the A & C populations to support the service users from within their respective communities. This includes the view that care and support should be made available in the communities, and the need for Black organisations to provide support that will promote treatment in the community. An example of this view is included in Leonie's statement in which she mentioned that organisations could be set up in the community to support service users experiencing mental health challenges to be supported by their peers, even to the extent that hospitalisation may not become necessary as a result of the community support they receive:

> *"The community could...I mean...systems could be erm.....organisation could be put in to place within the community. There could be more things within the community for people with difficulty or with mental health concerns to engage with others...peer....like peer support. To possibly strengthen our relationships and maybe even deter someone to getting too severe with their mental illness where they even have to be admitted in the first place"* (FG1).

The opening of community centres was also advocated by Jane, as she asserted that drop in services. In citing her experience as a client who has experience of ward visiting and peer support, she also stated that some people whom she had come across in hospitals were not supposed to have been hospitalised, as they were 'very misunderstood', and should have been provided support and received care in the community:

> *"If there were more drop-in services available to them, more services out in the community. Some of these people don't have to be in hospital I don't think, maybe I'm wrong but I don't think they do. They're just very misunderstood people these people"* (FG1).

A similar view in respect of the need for places to go and receive support in the community was also expressed by Alan, who indicated that there is a lack of such facilities in the community:

> *"I just, yes, somebody in the community. I'm always looking out for things, there's not much. You might have things*

> *there that you may be interested in you know that ... because if I'm at home what is there to do? You can't be too normal you know so....."* (1-1).

In highlighting the role of stigma of mental health challenges, Brian also suggested that individuals experiencing mental health challenges be treated in the community rather than in hospitals. He also mentioned the need to provide counselling in the community with the involvement of referral by their General Practitioners:

> *"By treating them in the communities, or going as far back as the GPs. Some people might not even need to come in to hospital. It's a stigma I feel because they are very misunderstood people. IF there were more services available to them in the community instead of putting them in a hospital setting. By starting off with the GPs, maybe they have issues; they might not even necessarily have mental health problems but it's the stigma of mental illness or whatever. They might not even be that ill that they have to be hospitalised. Ok get them to the GP and the GP might refer them for counselling"* (1-1).

The need for community organisations was also expressed from the context that there is more need for community organisations and drop in facilities rather than an increase in number of hospitals. An example of this view is contained in Patrick's statements in which he highlighted the need for support in the community to prevent mental illness as opposed to building more hospitals:

> *"It's investment. I don't know...re...re...re-organising the accounts so that some more can go into the community in order...as a preventative measure as opposed to investing in ....more within the hospital. They need to reach out and..and do more and you know this has been said for years but that's exactly what they need to do"* (FG1).

He also cited his observation that some community centers had been closed in certain communities and the need to open those centers with well paid staff as necessary tools for good services for improving Black mental health:

> *"Closing down all the centers and not wanting to pay staff in the community is not really incentive, is it? You know you need to have incentive, you need to have the right people in the right place to do the things that they most care about and have a genuine concern for the people who are attending or under their wing.* (Patrick, FG1).

Some participants also advocated for community action to promote discussions between the community members and the policy makers in respect of policies and procedures, and to encourage accountability of the services. Jane stated that members of the community can express their views to the NHS staff in respect of their policies, as well as seeking answers from the NHS on issues of concern:

> *"Well they need to talk, they need to talk because a lot their policies and procedures at NHS a lot of their umm.. a lot of their policies and procedures are made available to the public so perhaps the community might need to go into the trust and express that there is a need for something and allow the trust to explain themselves".* (FG1).

In line with this view, Brian also stated that the voices of the members of the community could be heard by setting up forums in the community, including support groups to enable 'voices be heard':

> *"By setting up some sort of a forum. Somebody has to start it up ... Like have some meetings and erm....maybe some sort of a support group, something like that...for those people and help them deal with the NHS, get some stuff. Let their voices be heard".* (FG1).

Also in line with the idea that the members of the community need to have some approach towards tackling the challenges of A & C mental health, Dwayne also highlighted the role of the NHS as a public body that also needs to provide 'assurances', and that the NHS should be asked to account to the community in respect to the services they provide. He advocates that the community needs to approach the services and highlight areas they feel that there is 'particular crisis' and 'people are suffering':

> *"They need to demonstrate and give assurances because it's a public body, it's not a private organisation so therefore people have to ...sometimes...what it...if the horse ..you can't force the horse to drink...something about water and horse. But sometimes you have to go in and say to the trust, you have to answer to this particular crisis because people are suffering".* (1-1).

In addition, within the perception of the role of 'communities', it was also expressed that the A & C community should also take action to support the young people by raising awareness about the likelihood of their behaviour being misunderstood by professionals in the public, which could lead to poor mental health experiences, including coercive pathways via the police and other services. Participants stated that as the over representation of the A & C and other BME individuals in mental health settings was in part due to the misunderstanding of the behaviours of the BME people, which, in turn, lead them to be arrested or sectioned for mental illness, it was expressed that education and awareness raising need to be undertaken to support young people. An example of this opinion is contained in Jane's statement in which she cited examples of young people 'getting picked up now', and expressed that awareness need to be raised for the younger generation regarding the likelihood of their behaviours being misunderstood and lead to hospitalisation via coercive pathways:

> *"Well we have to start educating our..our younger ones to say if you demonstrate certain things on the street people could interpret it in a negative way and it could be detrimental to you. So we have to start talking, we have to start helping the younger ones because they're the ones*

who are getting picked up now.....well...a lot of the time now and we have to start publicising that you know, different people do behave in different ways. The fact that you know this is a multi-racial society you know, we can't all be the same, we just can't. There are lots of things that have changed since I was a young girl and today. You know, for example like cueing up at the bus stop. When I was younger you had to cue, now people just surge on the bus and that's because of culture just saying "why are we cueing up? We wanna get on, let's get on" and you have to go with it because at the end of the day who is going to stand up and risk being harmed?" (FG1).

5.5.1. What Does This Mean For All Community Stakeholders?

The abovementioned contains the opinions of the participants in respect of what they perceive that community approaches need to be in order to address their concerns regarding the experiences of the A & C people with services. It includes their suggestions that support for mental health challenges should be made available by setting up community organisations to address the needs of the respective communities. This includes drop in centres as well as services that provide peer support and counselling for people within the communities.

The role of the community in expressing their views of services collectively through forums and other community groupings also seem to be highlighted as necessary to ensure that the NHS as a public body is made to listen to the concerns of the community and reflect their views in its policies, especially as it relates to the service experiences of the groups from the A & C communities. This seems to suggest that the setting up of community focused pressure groups are being advocated in order to raise issues of concern by the communities to the NHS, its policy makers and staff.

The emphasis on the word 'community' in the suggestions from the participants seems to indicate that they consider members of the A & C populations as a 'community'. Although the understanding of the concept of 'community' could be prone to subjective interpretations, it seems that this idea could have some link with the idea of collectivism (to which the BME peoples belong), and the idea that members of the collectivist society operate within the concept of community (Cheng et al, 2013). It also suggests that the externality in LOC found in the analysis of the views expressed by the majority of the participants in this study have resulted from a perception that the clients from the A & C populations are not being treated as members of a community by services, which, in turn, led to poor service experiences for the clients.

5.6. Clients Approaches – What People With Lived Experiences Of Mental Health Challenges Need To Do?

This final subtheme contains the opinions of the participants with respect to what they perceived as a need for the clients to also have inputs into changing their negative experiences they have expressed which contributed to their externality in mental health LOC.

In this respect, participants indicated that clients from the A & C populations also need to take some actions in order to improve the experiences they have commented on in their relationship with mental health services. This includes the need for clients to approach the mental health trusts by forming themselves into networks to raise issues of concern. One of the examples in this regard is contained in the suggestion by Bianca that networks can be set up by clients in the community with a view to approaching the trusts to raise their concerns:

> *"..they can ..they can approach the trust too. They can um...they can try to set up, they can try to set up networks in the community"* (1-1).

Noella also suggested clients getting together to set up meetings in order to identify common and individual needs by which they can also access support for them:

> *"I think kind of get together with people and kind of find out what individual people's needs are and kind of push....be more kind of vocal in kind of pushing forward in what you know some of the common needs are whether it be through these kind of meetings or whatever we had or you know the right place that needs to go and talk or making our individual needs kind of....well really kind of promoted"* (1-1).

The need for A & C clients to support one another was highlighted by Bianca, whilst indicating that this also has some challenges, including what she referred to as the added pressure of having to look after someone else, in peer support:

> *"They can try to support...support each other but it's hard work looking after...especially if you've got ill health yourself. Looking out for someone else can be quite pressurising for some people but that's why you need somebody there as overall support"* (1-1).

The foregoing indicates that the participants perceive that clients could also exert some control over their experiences with services by teaming together with other clients. The advantage of being more effective by approaching services in groups within the community also indicates the possible advantages of strength in number as well as the possibility of being able to achieve inclusion and peer support. It was also suggested that the effectiveness of such peer support arrangement could be enhanced if they were also received support.

5.7. Summary-Theme 5- What the Members Think

This section which focused on the suggestions by the participants on the way forward contains their opinions in respect of how they believed that the concerns they have raised could be addressed. Their suggestions have been divided into three approaches. They include the role of the services and health professionals, the role of the communities as well as the clients. They have indicated that the health services need to promote the recruitment of professionals from the A & C populations as well as into higher roles within the services. This is with a view to ensuring that professionals who understand the A & C culture are made to serve the service users, as well as to harness the impact of them acting as role models for people within the respective populations.

The health professionals who are not from the A & C backgrounds are also expected by the participants to show interest in the cultures of the people they serve, engage with them and embrace the knowledge of their cultures, including history and its impact on the health of the groups. The health professionals are also expected by the participants to be provided training on cultures of the minority groups in the community in order to increase their understanding of their needs (Bennett & Keating, 2009). Health professionals are also expected to listen and take into account the views of their clients from the A & C groups, their family members and friends, and include them in the decision making regarding their welfare, in order to ensure that they feel included and that their views are taken into consideration in the health care process, in order to promote internality in the service users' LOC, and achieve positive outcomes.

The community approaches advocated from the suggestions of the participants in this study include the perceived need to have services provided in the communities rather than in hospitals, the need to have community organisations set up to address the challenges of the respective A & C populations, by providing support inside these organisations, thereby providing community relapse support, counselling and reducing the need for hospitalisation. It also includes after discharge support, socialisation and peer support. Community groups could also be set up as pressure groups to approach the NHS to raise issues of concern in respect of the services they receive and with a view to seeking improvement in the experiences of the A & C groups with services.

The client inputs advocated in this report also includes setting up forums and groups by clients to support one another as well as to present their concerns to services as members of groups of clients, in order to improve service experiences.

The abovementioned indicates that the participants in this study believe that the service experiences can be improved if the three-pronged approaches they have recommended are put in place. This seems to corroborate the importance of the need for A & C service users being organised into supporting their members in voluntary sector settings (Campbell, 2004).

Part II

Introduction: A brief about what this part covers

This part of the book contains what you could consider as theoretical aspects of the study. It includes a background on the status of the Mental Health of Black and Minority Ethnic peoples in the United Kingdom, the research concepts, processes, and procedures.

1 | Background, Aims and Objectives of the Study

> *"Patients from Black or Black British ethnic groups appear to be more highly represented .... suggesting the pathways into mental health care are different for Black and ethnic minority patients. Such adverse pathways could be a result of inequalities in access to, or outcomes from mental health services, even if this is a reflection of different service provision in different areas of the country"* (Care Quality Commission, 2014:22).

This chapter explains the motivation and provides a rationale behind the study of African and Caribbean mental health experiences within the context of Black and Minority Ethnic (BME) mental health. This study focuses on A & C mental health service users specifically, but there will be a discussion of mental health in relation to the BME populations, as indicated in the quote from Care Quality Commission (2014) above. It contains an introduction into the main problem identified including the challenges in the mental health profile of the study population in the United Kingdom, including pathways, quality of care and negative outcomes. It also explores the concepts of Race, Ethnicity and Culture, including definitions and their relationship with the profiles of the BME and A & C service users. By focussing specially on the experiences of groups of African or Caribbean descent, it highlights the limitations of research to date and the identified gap in understanding relating to locus of control in their experiences with mental health services which has prompted this research, the interest of the author in the subject matter, as well as the aims and objectives of this study.

The mental health profile and concerns of Black and Minority Ethnic (BME) populations in England and the United Kingdom has been a subject of interest in the past decades (DoH, 2010; Care Quality Commission, 2014). This includes the over-representation of BME populations in psychiatric health care settings particularly for the African and Caribbean (A & C) communities (Care Quality Commission, CQC, 2014; Crisp et al, 2016; Keating, 2016). This is characterised by:

- Adverse entry pathways to services, including a comparatively higher level of police involvement and higher levels of admission by detention via the use of the Mental Health Act (MHA), (1983, 2007);
- Higher levels of coercive practices, including the over-use of the MHA (2007) in seclusion and restraints (Keating, 2016; Bhui, et al, 2003);
- Over-use of medication, less focus on recovery approaches, and inequality in access to psychological therapies (Bhui, et al, 2003; Robinson et al, 2011; Keating, 2012; Adebowale, 2013);
- Poorer outcomes and adverse results, in comparison with other ethnic minorities and their white counterparts in the United Kingdom (Keating et al, 2002; Morgan et al, 2004; Edge et al, 2016). Adverse results include death involving A & C clients in services due to the use of restraint (Norfolk, Suffolk and Cambridgeshire Strategic Health Authority, 2003; Bradby, 2010);
- A high dissatisfaction rate in their experiences with mental health services, including perceived adverse stereotypes, such as being Black and dangerous (Bhui, et al, 2003; Robinson et al, 2011; Keating, 2012; Adebowale, 2013; Mantovani et al, 2017; Centre for Mental Health, CMH, 2017);
- These experiences sometimes culminate in avoidance of and resistance to Mental Health Services (MHS) (Mantovani et al, 2017; Kotecha, 2008), and late entry to services, which combine to promote the circles of fear. This issue was highlighted in the 'Breaking the circles of fear' report by

Keating et al (2002), which found that members from the A & C groups experienced fear of mental health services;

- Their experiences have been characterised by a lack of awareness, acknowledgement, and consideration of their culture by professionals and services, which combine with other challenges to exacerbate the inequality in outcomes (Keating & Robertson, 2004; DoH, 2013).

The above factors are further expanded upon in Addendum 1 below, which was originally added as an appendix in the thesis (The challenge of disparities in mental health involving BME communities), including rates of disparities in mental illness involving these groups, schizophrenia diagnosis, treatment, and care outcomes, (CQC, 2011; 2014); increase in number of BME people who died in custody due to mental illness related incidences (Independent Police Complaints Commission, ((IPCC), 2012; Adebowale, 2013). It also includes the Chief Medical Officer's report relating to decisions being made by health professionals and services without awareness and consideration for the 'cultural origins of the patient, let alone showing awareness of how professional cultures and systems of care impact on clinical decision-making.' (DoH, 2013: 276); and the contribution of the lack of cultural awareness to discrimination on account of culture, misdiagnosis and poor care, to the over-representation and inequalities (Keating et al, 2002; McKenzie &Bhui, 2007).

1.1. Addendum 1- The Challenge of Disparities in Mental Health Involving BME Communities

It has been acknowledged that achieving good mental health care for individuals from BME communities is one of the biggest challenges for mental health services in England and Wales (Commission for Healthcare Audit and Inspection, 2005; NHS, 2016) because the disparities in rates of mental illness such as schizophrenia, treatment, care and outcomes persist (CQC, 2011; 2014); comparatively lower level of primary care entry to services, higher level through the police and the criminal justice system (Borschmann et al, 2010; CQC, 2011) .

Studies into incidences of psychosis for migrant populations in the UK have also reported comparatively higher levels for Black populations, especially Caribbean and Black African populations, than the mainstream populations (Moffat et al, 2009; Bhui et al, 2014; Edge, 2016). In addition to the finding by Fernando (1998) that incidences of Schizophrenia diagnosis were high for African Caribbean people in England in relation to cultural implications, a major study titled *'Aetiology and Ethnicity of Schizophrenia and Other Psychoses (AESOP)'* carried out between 1997 and 1999 found that:

> *"Psychosis incidence was higher in all British ethnic minority groups than in the White British group .... Schizophrenia and mania were highest in African-Caribbeans (schizophrenia incidence per 100 000 persons per year: 70.7 in African-Caribbeans vs 7.2 in White British; incidence rate ratio (IRR) 9.1, 95% CI 6.6 to 12.6; mania incidence per 100 000 persons per year: 15.5 in African-Caribbeans vs 2.2 in White British; IRR 8.0, 95% CI 4.3 to 14.8), and second highest in Black-Africans (schizophrenia incidence per 100 000 persons per year: 40.3; IRR vs White British: 5.8, 95% CI 3.9 to 8.4; mania incidence per 100 000 persons per year: 12.3; IRR vs White British: 6.2, 95% CI 3.1 to 12.1)"* (Fearon et al, 2007:95).

This result has also been highlighted as indicative that migrant populations are susceptible to psychosis and misdiagnosis, with the consequent need to provide services that are suitable for their needs (Cantor-Graae, 2007).

The experiences of members of A & C communities with mental health challenges have also been characterised by a high rate of detention and use of coercive measures in mental health settings, and low level of referral through primary care; as BME groups do not normally enter the MHS via their local General Practitioners but through the Police (Section 136 of the MHA 1983) and criminal justice system (Borschmann et al, 2010; Care Quality Commission, 2011). The

Chief Medical Officer report (Department of Health, DoH, 2013: 276) also highlights "differing pathways to care, less use of primary care, difficulties in being diagnosed early, communications of distress that were not recognised by professionals, more hospital admissions (for black Caribbean and black African groups), less psychotherapy and more somatic interventions".

The report by the Care Quality Commission (2011) which reported the results of the 2010 *Count mein* national census of inpatients and patients on supervised community treatment in mental health and learning disability services in England and Wales, reported "a 'consistent pattern' of higher detention rates under Section 37/41 for Black Caribbean and Other Black groups across all six of the annual censuses" (Adebowale, 2013:37). This situation persists even though the needs, issues and concerns of Black and minority ethnic groups with mental health problems were at the fore of the Government policy agenda (DoH, 2003; DoH, 2005; Bradley, 2009; Care Quality Commission, 2011).

Statistics have also indicated that nearly half (seven out of fifteen) of individuals who died either whilst in police custody or following detention by the police in 2011/2012 were due to mental illness (Independent Police Complaints Commission, (IPCC), 2012). The proportion of persons from the BME populations who have died in this circumstance rose from 32 per cent in 2009 to 38% in 2011 (IPCC, 2012; Adebowale, 2013).

The report by the Care Quality Commission, CQC, (2014:12) on the use of the MHA for 2012/2013 indicated that "...as in previous years, showed a continuing trend in high rates of detention among certain black and minority ethnic groups".

The chart by CQC (2014: 21) below (*Figure 1- Mental Health Act Use by Ethnicity, 2012/13*) indicates that if the level of expected detention relative to size of the population is 100, different groups are variously more or less frequently detained than expected, but the African, Caribbean and Other Black groups recorded the highest rates.

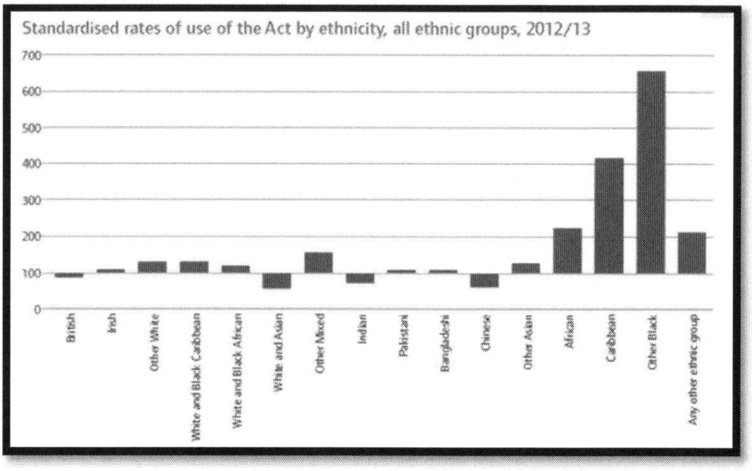

Figure 1: Mental Health Act Use by Ethnicity, 2012/13
Source: Monitoring the Mental Health Act in 2012/13. Care Quality Commission (2014).
http://www.cqc.org.uk/sites/default/files/documents/cqc_mentalhealth_2012_13_07_update.pdf

A more recent report from the independent Mental Health Taskforce to the NHS in England (2016) stated that "Men of African and Caribbean heritage are up to 6.6 times more likely to be admitted as inpatients or detained under the Mental Health Act, indicating a systemic failure to provide effective crisis care for these groups" (NHS, 2016: 9).

The absence of improvement on previous statistics was further highlighted by the CQC in the same report that "Detention rates were particularly high for, Black African (2.2 times higher), Black Caribbean (4.2 times higher), Other Black (6.6 times higher) and other groups (2.1 times higher)" (CQC, 2014:20). This indicates that there was no recorded improvement to previous years in the over representation of BME groups in relation to the rate of detention.

Awareness, acknowledgement, and consideration of cultural issues have also been observed as a problem in the inequality in outcomes and experience of BME groups in mental health (Keating &

Robertson, 2004; DoH, 2013). This was also indicated in the Chief Medical Officer report (DoH, 2013:276) that “These inequalities of experience and outcome have been understood in terms of clinicians behaving differently and making decisions that are not fully cognisant of the cultural origins of the patient, let alone showing awareness of how professional cultures and systems of care impact on clinical decision-making”. This suggests that the absence of recognition of cultural differences and needs of the BME patients are likely to have contributed to discrimination on account of culture, misdiagnosis and poor care, which could ultimately have contributed to the over representation of the BME populations in health care settings (Keating et al, 2002; McKenzie & Bhui, 2007).

2| The Contested Natures of Race, Ethnicity and Culture

Race has been described as a term that relates to 'ancestry, descent, and heredity', and seen as a characteristic of human genetics (Ballard, 2002: 2). It has been observed that race as a concept was said to have been first introduced into 'biological literature' by Buffon in 1749, which was 'explicitly regarded as an arbitrary classification, serving only as a convenient label and not a definable scientific entity' (Agyemang et al, 2005: 1014).

Ballard (2002) asserted that race is also used to highlight supposed categorical differences between different sub-sections of humans, in which case race can be considered in the context of the human race 'such as 'the European race', the 'African race''(Ballard, 2002: 3). It was also stressed by Ballard (2002), that the social connotations of the two perspectives, one referring to humanity while the other refers to subdivisions are mirror images of one another. Whilst the first underlines common humanity, the second suggests that there are indisputable differences between different subsections of humanity (Ballard, 2002).

The biological assumption behind race that relies on differences in skin colour and other physical characteristics, for example, eye colour, hair colour, have led to notions of superiority and inferiority. It has also been observed to have been historically used as a tool for differentiation, racism, a claim of superiority of groups to others and other political ends (David & Cooper, 1986). David and Cooper (1986) also asserted that differences in human beings are not in 'discrete' forms but are more of social and environmental factors than genetics.

It has also been observed that the error in the biological basis of race lies in the fact that various differences do not only exist within groups categorised as being of 'same race' but these differences are seen to be greater than the differences found to exist between groups categorised as being of 'different races' (Agyemang et al, 2005). This has been referred to as the existence of "more genetic variation within than between groups" (Agyemang et al, 2005:1014). Rathwell and Phillips (1986) also observed that race was synonymous with skin colour, which was not helpful in relation to health, as "there are as many physiological and health variations occurring amongst persons with the same skin colouring as between colours."(Rathwell& Phillips, 1986:1) The impact of the conceptualisation of race based on biology has also been highlighted in Fernando's (2010) assertion that this conceptualisation of race that relies on making references to differences in types of human bodies only acts as significant symbols of social and cultural divisions and conflicts in the society. The concept of race should, therefore, not be a biological construct but a social one, whereby individuals are belonging to social groupings rather than putting them into categories based on their physical features.

Race can also be considered alongside ethnicity as 'social constructions, with different individual and social meanings according to the context in which they are applied' (Robinson et al, 2011:83). Indeed, the word 'race' has also been referred to in apostrophe (Craig et al, 2012), due to the position that "it is a social construct with particular historical connotations with no objective meaning" (Craig et al, 2012: xiii). It has also been stated that racial groups within this social context of categorisation should be the basis by which individuals' health needs should be considered and addressed as quoted above (David & Cooper, 1986).

This social constructionist view of 'race', which posits that skin colour and other physical features do not indicate differences in biological make up and should not be used as the basis for categorising individuals into groups (Fernando, 2009; Machery & Faucher, 2005), is the basis on which the participants of this study has been defined. This means that they are identified by the way they describe themselves socially, as members of A & C populations; this may not necessarily be defined by their physical features (Fernando, 2009), but by their self-described social grouping and countries of origin. They are, therefore, made up of individuals whose parents and/or grandparents migrated to the United Kingdom from Africa and the Caribbean.

Ethnicity has been described by Agyemang et al, (2012: 1014) as a multidimensional concept which encompasses one or more "shared origins or social backgrounds; shared culture or tradition that are distinctive, maintained between generations, and lead to a sense of identity and group; and a common language or religious tradition". These characteristics dictate behaviour, cultural practices, norms and values of groups, which may, in turn, combine with environmental factors to determine health outcomes or profiles (Agyemang et al, 2012). The original word 'ethnic' was said to have originated from the Greek word 'ethnos', which generally implied 'people living together; a tribe, nation, caste' which 'could be used to exclude groups.' (Craig et al, 2012: 23). Ethnicity has also been described as "a subjective impression of how groups see themselves. It is an ambiguous term in that one's ethnicity may be different according to context and change from time to time" (Fernando & Keating, 2009: 17). These dynamics are, however, fluid in nature as they are changeable over time and in different contexts and depend on the way individuals identify themselves with specific groups.

Ethnicity has also been observed to be different from ethnic origin, which is like one's race (Agyemang et al, 2012; Craig et al, 2012). This, in turn, indicates that someone may belong to a specific ethnicity but chose not to identify themselves with such ethnic group due to changes over time, the context, or their own choice of preferences (Agyemang et al, 2012; Craig et al, 2012).

The fluidity in ethnicity has also been highlighted in relation to culture and context (Hall, 1993). For example, it has been observed that groups may respond to experience of racism by either choosing to identify with other groups based on religion or places of their birth. Groups of different backgrounds could also choose to group together based on race, for example as 'Black', which often includes 'non-Black'

(Fernando & Keating, 2009). The importance of this has been highlighted as many persons could be placed within specific groups by other groups based on their understanding or assumption of their ethnicity or ethnic groupings, which could be flawed (Fernando, 2009). For example, as there are multiple islands in the Caribbean (Agyemang et al, 2012); the second or third generations of individuals who migrated from the Caribbean but who were born in the UK may choose not to self-identify themselves as Caribbean, depending on the contexts in which they are asked, although someone else could choose to group such individuals as Caribbean. This suggests the existence of a notion of multiple or interchangeable identities (Hall, 1993).

This indicates categorising individuals into groups based on some specific stereotypes or physical characteristics without considering the context, and without liaising with the individuals and clarifying such categorisation, are likely to lead to flawed understanding and consequent actions or health interventions (Craig et al, 2012). Ethnicity also been referred to within the context of an absence of clarity in conceptualising ethnic diversity and differences in the United Kingdom, which, in turn, can lead to confusion in relation to policy and guidelines relating to health and social care (Craig et al, 2012: 4). In observing for example that there is silence in acknowledgement of ethnicities in the 'White' groups, it has also been observed that policy and practice 'rarely acknowledge that everyone has an ethnicity' (Craig et al, 2012: 4).

Culture has been defined as "'conceptual structures'-a flexible system of values and worldviews that groups live by, define their identities by and negotiate their lives by" (Fernando & Keating, 2009: 16). Hall (1993) quoted Williams' definition of culture in The Long Revolution (1961), as 'a description of a particular way of life which expresses certain meanings and values, not only in art and learning, but in institutions and ordinary behaviour' (Hall, 1993: 351). Culture also encompasses the way by which individuals conceptualise their own way of life and how they relate to one another. Culture has also been attributed to fluidity and flexibility, relates to language, heritage, values, religion and religious practices, traditions, modes of dressing, food, and views about the world (Fernando & Keating, 2009).

The importance of the fluid nature of cultures, the likelihood that individuals can identify with other groups or specific groups for different reasons and at different times also highlights the error that may arise in stereotyping individuals or grouping them based on physical features such as skin colour or observed religious affiliations. For example, it has been observed that groups of individuals of minority ethnic backgrounds in the UK are treated by state institutions as "undifferentiated collectives of (metaphorical and literal) 'immigrants'" (Craig et al, 2012: 20). This has led to them being "defined through stereotypes of culture, religion and tradition, rather than as citizens in their own right negotiating their multiple identities differently within specific social and political contexts" (Craig et al, 2012: 20-21). Consequently, inequality in healthcare has also been attributed to be promoted by the phenomenon of subjective homogenous grouping of persons without due consideration for individual differences or preferences in different or similar contexts (Craig et al, 2012).

2.1. Ethnicity, Race, Culture – Implications for BME Mental Health

The definitions of race, ethnicity and culture have also been explored in the context of their implications for mental health (Fernando & Keating, 2009; McKenzie &Bhui, 2007). As has been noted earlier, race and ethnicity are the concepts that can be applied as tools to place individuals into groups along racial, religious, cultural and ethnic lines (Fernando, 2010). In relation to mental health, it has been posited that a different approach needs to be taken to view these concepts, in contrast to the notion that the appreciation of the concepts be based on the definitions given to them (Fernando & Keating, 2009). It has, thus, been argued that "'race' and 'ethnicity' should be viewed as social constructs, with different individual and societal meanings depending on the context in which they are applied" (Keating, 2012: 210). This is since ethnicity, culture along with racism carry 'negative social meanings', especially for Black and Minority

Ethnic (BME) groups in the UK, as they intersect "with other issues which constitute social divisions in the society including age, ability, class, gender, and sexuality" (Keating, 2012: 210).

It has also been observed that creating stereotypes of specific races, especially Black peoples in the UK has promoted racism, which has, in turn, led to mental health difficulties for the BME individuals (Keating, 2012). For example, the notions of aggression and dangerousness, have impacted on the Black men's mental health profile, as it was also observed that "for African and Caribbean men, being seen as 'big, black, bad, dangerous and mad' (Keating, 2012: 214) can lead to conceptions that they are less deserving of treatment that would lead them to pathways of recovery" (Keating, 2012: 214). This has been attributed to the decision to apply containment, sedation approaches rather than therapeutic interventions (Keating, 2012). The connection of 'race, madness and dangerousness' has also been identified to be a stimulus in constructing identities of Black peoples (Keating, 2016). A recent report referred to statistics indicates that the rate of inequalities in outcomes in relation to mental health have not improved, as the rate of detention of Black groups in the UK under the Mental health Act continue to rise (CMH, 2017; NHS, 2017). For example, the latest report by NHS England (2017) indicates that "detention rates for the 'Black or Black British' group (272.1 detentions per 100,000 population) were highest, over four times those of the White group (67.0 per 100,000 population), which was lowest" (NHS, 2017: 11).

Some of the other disadvantages that have emanated as consequences of the social divisions along racial, cultural and/or ethnic lines in the UK include racism, over representation of BME groups in mental health settings, comparatively higher diagnosis of schizophrenia amongst A & C groups, the 'circles of fear' (Edge, 2011) of not seeking help for mental health issues by African and Caribbean groups, less likelihood of Caribbean women seeking help for perinatal depression, and social deprivation which impacts on mental health (Keating & Robertson, 2004; Keating, 2012; Edge, 2011; Mantovani et al, 2017).

The relationship between the experiences of the Caribbean population, their migration into the United Kingdom and its association with mental health issues have also been highlighted (Miranda et al, 2005. For example, it has been underlined that:

> *"Immigrant populations from the Caribbean are found to have higher rates of depression than do those in the British general population" (Miranda et al, 2005: 257).*

It has also been highlighted that "persistent stereotypes and coupling of dangerousness with Black men and strength with Black women results in resources being disproportionately directed towards coercive treatment of Black British Caribbean men in secondary and tertiary psychiatric services at the expense of primary care interventions and women's mental health in this group" (Edge, 2013: 44). This further highlights the view that these concepts can be used as tools to segregate persons into groups to foster inequality and discrimination against minority groups.

A major finding in relation to these definitions and perspectives within which they are defined lies in the suggestion that self-description should be the key to how individuals are considered, especially for research purposes that relate to ethnicity, as individuals may experience a sense of disconnect with their identity (Agyemang et al, 2005). Research should, therefore, be based on how individuals perceive themselves, their sense of shared culture or ethnicity, values, and norms in relation to other groups. This is in order to prevent flawed generalisations which could ultimately lead to false or inaccurate depiction or results. For example, in a study related to exploring ethnicity, gender and mental health (Robinson, Keating & Robertson, 2011: 82), the subjects of the study were chosen from men 'who describe themselves as belonging to a minority group in the UK, with a shared ethnicity and language and/or culture'. In another study in relation to perinatal mental health care (Edge, 2011: 257), majority of the subjects of the study were women who 'were born in the UK but self-labelled as being 'of black Caribbean origin'.

In summary, this section has explored the meaning of ethnicity, race and culture, including the various perspectives within which the discourses of the concepts have become popular. It also includes the demonstration of the fact that these three concepts are not only contested constructs but are interrelated. They are also mostly politically, personally and socially constructed to suit various interests. In the light of these observations, the focuses of this study were based on the participants who self-described themselves as African or Caribbean.

2.2. Terminology of Use- Black, African, Caribbean-Descriptions of African and Caribbean Groups In Health Research

2.2.1. BME and African Caribbean- Terminology

Several debates have emerged regarding the terminology used in describing groups with ancestral origins from the Caribbean as well as those from the African continent (Agyemang et al, 2005). It has been observed that this continues to pervade although there are observed differences in migration history, language, culture, beliefs, values, diet, customs, and other issues between African Caribbean groups and other African populations (Agyemang et al, 2005). The complexity of the historical backgrounds of groups who migrated from the Caribbean to Great Britain was highlighted by Arnold (2012) in which it was observed that one set of migrants was made up of descendants of those who were referred to as 'West Indians' by Christopher Columbus in 1492, who originated from the islands and the two mainland territories of the erstwhile British colonies in the Caribbean region.

Another set arose from the many Black groups in Britain who subsequently chose to be called 'African Caribbean' (Arnold, 2012), having described themselves as different from the native Caribbean but identified themselves as progenies of Africans who were taken by Europeans to the Caribbean during the slavery era. Attempts have also been made to provide some definitions and guides for ease of understanding. This includes the glossary that centred "on the concepts and terminology used in the study of the health of minority ethnic and racial groups" (Bhopal, 2004: 441).

This glossary defined persons of Afro-Caribbean or African Caribbean as, "A person of African ancestral origins whose family settled in the Caribbean before emigrating and who self identifies, or is identified, as Afro-Caribbean" (Bhopal, 2004: 443). In the same glossary, Bhopal describes the term African as "A person with African ancestral origins who self identifies, or is identified, as African, but excluding those of other ancestry, for example, European and South Asian." The British Sociological Association's (2005) guidelines which "were originally drawn up by the BSA Black Women's Sub-Committee and revised by the BSA Race Forum" (BSA, 2005:1) indicated that "African-Caribbean has replaced the term Afro-Caribbean to refer to Caribbean groups and those of Caribbean origin who are of African descent. There is now a view that the term should not be hyphenated and that indeed, the differences between such groups mean the groups of A & C origins should be referred to separately" (BSA, 2005: 1).

The BSA referred to the basis of its guidelines as the "common uses of these terms in everyday language and by social scientists while writing about ethnicity and race" (BSA, 2005:1). However, it has been observed that the two groups continued to be combined by health researchers despite the recognition of the differences between Caribbean groups by the Census in the United Kingdom (Agyemang et al, 2005: 1016).

On the other hand, studies involving groups whose families migrated to the United Kingdom from Africa are termed as Black African (Agyemang et al, 2005: 1016). This term has also been described "as usually used in the UK, refers to groups and their offspring with African ancestral origins who migrated via sub-Saharan Africa. The term has a geographical meaning and a more general one". Agyemang et al, (2005) also observed that the suitability of the term Black African has also been challenged by groups whose families originated from the parts of Africa that were presumed to share commonalities with Arabic cultures. In the same vein people termed Africans are persons" with African ancestral origins who self identifies or is identified by others as Africans, but usually excludes those residents of Africa of other ancestry, for example, Europeans and South Asians and sometimes excludes North Africans, for example, Algerians" (Agyemang et al, 2005:1017). This suggests also that there is a need to indicate the specific part of Africa the persons originated from; there is also a tendency for them to be categorised as Caribbean by joining them with groups of Caribbean origin.

It has been posited that studies conducted in Europe and North America that relate to people who had African ancestral heritages and migrated through the islands of the Caribbean have used several titles to describe the study participants; the terms include African Caribbean, Afro-Caribbean, (Agyemang et al, 2005). In citing some examples of general health studies in the UK, Agyemang et al (2005), however, observed that inconsistency of use of these terms has pervaded in the United Kingdom. This includes Cruickshank et al, (1991) and Karlsen et al, (2001) who used the terms African Caribbean and Afro-Caribbean to refer to groups of Black and Caribbean origins. Other examples include Cappuccio et al, (1998); Chaturvedi & McKeigue, (1993), and Haines et al (1987), who used the same terms to refer to groups of either West African or Caribbean descent.

A similarity has also been found in more recent studies and reports in the United Kingdom, as several health and social care related studies have predominantly referred to peoples of A & C ethnic origins and ancestry by using various terminologies. Some examples include 'African Caribbean' (Fearon et al, 2006; Robinson et al, 2011); 'Afro Caribbean' (The National Institute for Mental Health in England, 2008); 'African and African-Caribbean' (Campbell, 2004; Morgan et al, 2005; Gupta & Featherstone, 2015; Kalathil, 2011); 'Black Caribbean' (Crisp et al, 2016), 'Black British Caribbean (Edge, (2013); 'Black' (Gupta & Featherstone, 2015); and 'Black Caribbean' (Edge, & Rogers, 2005; Edge, 2008, 2010, 2007). Some other studies relied on the 2001 Census in the UK to describe groups who were born in the Caribbean, or whose family originated in the Caribbean as African Caribbean (Fearon et al, 2006; Campbell, 2004). This was like the way in which groups who were born in or whose family originated from sub-Saharan Africa were referred to in the Census as Black African (Agyemang et al (2005). A more recent study relating to mental health stigma and BME has jointly referred to the groups as "African-descended groups in the UK (primarily people with origins in Africa and the Caribbean)" (Mantovani et al, 2017: 374).

2.3. Terminology of Use- Implications for This Book

The implication of the existence of the different terminologies used lies in the need for researchers to recognise and acknowledge the heterogeneity of A & C populations and that their "lived experiences are differentiated by their histories, cultures, ethnicities and social circumstances" (Bernard and Gupta, 2008: 2). In the light of the potential confusion emanated from the terminology used for study participants in minority health studies as observed in the preceding section, it has been decided that this study relied on the definition of the A & C participants based on the following principles:

- The subjects of this thesis were based on the participants who self-described as African or Caribbean.
- The term 'Caribbean' was used to refer to the participants whose family originated from the Caribbean, including those with origins in Africa
- The term 'African' was used to describe the participants whose family originated from sub-Saharan Africa.
- No effort was made to distinguish between the self-described Caribbean participants from those whose descendants originated from the 'West Indian' category and those whose families originated from the African descendants' category as indicated earlier in this section (Arnold, 2012). This is, since majority of the participants were born in the United Kingdom and described as Black British and was not likely to be aware of the differences in categories, due to generational differences.
- No effort was made to differentiate the African participants by the location of their respective countries in Africa. This is due

to the similar issue with the Caribbean participants in respect of generational differences, as many of them were also born in the United Kingdom. However, majority of the participants who self-described as being of African origin informed the researcher that their parents and grandparents were born in countries in West Africa, including Nigeria and Ghana.

3| What Is Locus of Control as a Concept?

3.1. Introduction

A conceptual framework shows how research fits into what is already known, including the relationship to existing theory and inquiry (Maxwell, 2005). It also illustrates how research contributes on the topic to the field of investigation and informs the questions to be used for the study. A conceptual framework also guides the methodology and helps to justify problem being investigated, thereby highlighting the importance of the research (Schram, 2003; Maxwell, 2005). It has been summarised by Maxwell (2005), as "the system of concepts, assumptions, expectations, beliefs, and theories that support and inform your research". Maxwell (2005: 33).

This section explores the literature on LOC in this study, including its meaning, origin, and its applicability to various contexts, measurement and measuring scales, its applicability to health in general, mental health, and its relationship to culture and ethnicity with particular reference to the BME community in general and the A & C communities in particular. The relationship between LOC and collectivist and individualist cultures; the relationship between LOC and its relevance to mental health, the health seeking behaviours in mental health clients in general and those from the Black and Ethnic Minority (BME) community in particular; and the implications for provision and response to mental health services and social care are also explored. The rationale for applying LOC as a conceptual model and its applicability to this study in the context of its relationship with the culture of A & C peoples in mental health settings are also included.

<u>3.1.1. LOC Origin, Definition and Contextual Relevance</u>

> *"A sense of control is typically associated with better physical and emotional health; improved coping with*

> *stressful situations; and more successful behaviour and performance... Conversely, a loss of control often results in poor personal outcomes, as repeatedly illustrated by residents of institutions such as hospitals ... schools, and homes for the elderly"* (Ruggiero & Taylor, 1997: 375).

Locus of Control (LOC) describes how one personally evaluates reasons that explain events and results (Hill & Bale, 1980; Wood & Letak, 1982; Ruggiero and Taylor, 1997; Cheng et al., 2013). Rooted in psychology and social learning theories (Rotter, 1966; Bandura, 1977; Ogunyemi, 2013), LOC is based on how individuals conduct subjective appraisals of the factors that they perceive are responsible for the actions in their lives. LOC refers to the level to which individuals consider that they are able to influence their environment, and the extent to which the things that they experience or their fortunes are dictated by forces outside themselves, or circumstances beyond their control, including actions of other people and chance occurrences (Poortinga, et al, 2008; Tigani, et al, 2011). As indicated in (*Figure 2-Internal and External LOC*) below, LOC can be either internal or external. Internal LOC refers to a belief by an individual that events, occurrences and outcomes are decided by their own actions, while someone with an external LOC considers that their fortunes or otherwise are dictated by forces outside themselves, and for which they have little control or influence (Wood &Letak, 1982; Declerck et al, 2006; Poortinga, et al, 2008). This implies that they perceive that their actions would bear little or no relevance or make a difference to whatever happens to them. Social learning theorists including Rotter, (1966, 1975) and Bandura, (1977) assert that the way people perceive their sense of judgement over control in their lives are not inborn, but emanate from their individual experiences over time including effects from the society, which tend to strengthen their perception (Dijkstraa et al, 2011).

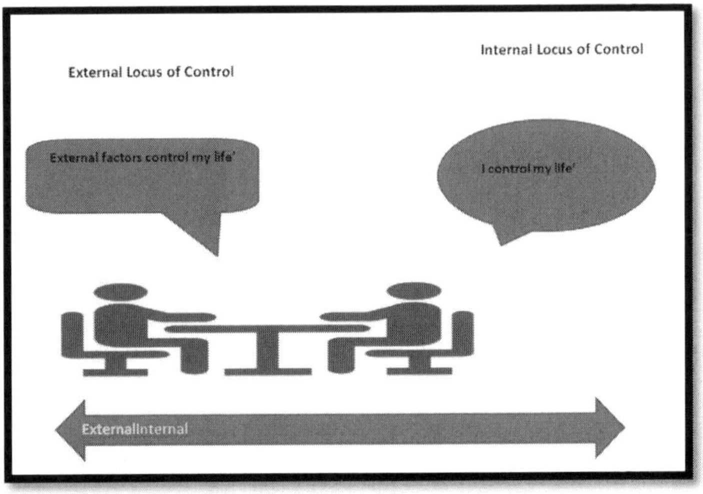

Figure 2: Internal and External LOC

This, in turn, becomes reinforced by various factors including their personality traits, their learning as well as how things are conducted in the society they belong (McDevitt et al., 2007). This leads to what has been termed generalised expectancies which, in turn, dictates human behaviour (Kasilingam & Sudha, 2010), that are subsequently reinforced psychologically, depending on situations. It is also suggested that what one generally expects would define one's behaviour, which, in turn, brings the concept of behaviour versus rewards (Kasilingam & Sudha, 2010). In other words, if one expects that one's behaviour is not likely to result in a change of circumstance or situation, or something positive or desired outcome, one is not likely to undertake such behaviour, just as what one expects as a result of behaviour will be the driver for such behaviours (Ryan & Francis, 2010). Peterson and Stunkard (1989) align with this position and stress that the extent to which one perceives control has a positive correlation with the level of motivation, managing with, and decrease of, pressure, and the resultant life style improvements (Ponto, 2004). Suizzo and Soon (2006) observed that an individual would develop a sense of internal LOC when they have observed over time that their actions have impacted on their environment rather than the other way round. On the other hand, an observed failure or perceived lack of impact on the environment or social interactions over time tends to lead an individual to develop an external orientation to Locus of Control, which may, in turn, lead them to choose to exert no effort to influence his environment, as they are likely to find such an exercise non-worthwhile (Adams et al, 2008).

3.2.2. Measurement of LOC

Research into LOC since the 1960s has evolved and consisted of efforts aimed at measuring LOC, beginning from the I-E measuring scales developed by Rotter (1966) titled "Generalized expectancies for internal versus external control of reinforcement". The scale was designed based on thirteen sets of dual statements from which the participant is expected to pick the statement that best describes how they feel and from which the responses are subjected to a scoring system designed by Rotter, which ranges from 0 to 13. A high score indicates an external locus of control while a low score indicates an internal locus of control (Rotter, 1966).

Levenson (1974) differed in opinion from Rotter's assertion, by indicating that internal and external LOC should not be treated as mutually exclusive. Other subsequent generalised scales have been developed using the Rotter Internal-External (I-E) Scale as the foundational basis to address specific areas. The development of these scales was aimed to highlight the existence of several control variables for which the individual may have very little influence over. These include those controls exerted by chance, fate and luck, which represented forces that does not follow a pattern, while the concept of powerful others including government establishments are seen as sources of control which could be subject to pattern (Levenson (1974; Paulus 1983; Lachman, 1986; Poortinga, et al, 2008).

This is in line with the thoughts of subsequent researchers who acknowledged that the LOC offers an opportunity to explore several dimensions of human behaviour and life, and have resulted in multidimensional instruments (Lefcourt, 1981; Paulus 1983; Lachman,

1986; Cheng et al, 2013). It was found that one is subject to various control variables which include the influence of others, chance and the individual personality traits. These variables tend to impact on the individual in different ways and degrees. Paulus, 1985 asserts that these control variables could impact on the person either in specific areas or domains of life or behaviour (Paulus, 1985; Lachman, 1986; Declerck et al, 2006).

LOC has also been described as a spectrum between internal and external into which most individuals can be found, and explains the fact that everyone, naturally, falls somewhere in between and within this spectrum. Their position within the spectrum is determined by the generalised expectancy that, in turn, influences the person's consequent conduct or behaviour (Hampson, 1995; Ponto, 2004; Cheng et al, 2013). Because of this, it has been agreed that one of the ways by which one could decipher the Locus of Control is by scale measurement (Declerck et al, 2006).

3.2.3. LOC Exploration in Non-Health Contexts

LOC has been a subject explored in various areas of human endeavour, behaviour and response since it was originated in the 1960s, including both health and non-health contexts. A study by Judge and Bono (2001) found a total of 9,339 articles citing LOC in PsycINFO database between 1967 and 1999. Some of the studies explored the relationship between LOC and type A behaviour pattern (Furnham, 1983); ageing research (Lachman, 1986); communication and public speaking (Hamilton, 1991); minority group's perception and minimisation of discrimination (Ruggiero & Taylor, 1997); job performance (Hough, 1992); job satisfaction and job performance (Judge & Bono, 2001); and leadership (Ogunyemi, 2013).

In highlighting the importance of perception of control, Ruggiero and Taylor, (1997) cited several studies which explored psychological theories, and articulated that several variables such as "control, efficacy, mastery, competence, and autonomy. For example, reactance theory (Brehm, 1972; Brehm & Brehm, 1981); the locus of control concept (Rotter, 1966); self-efficacy (Bandura, 1977, 1982,

1986); and the illusion of control (Langer, 1975)". Ruggiero and Taylor, (1997:375) conclude that all these "converge to suggest that perceived control is a desirous state that individuals are motivated to achieve".

In a study by O'Leary & Drabman, (1971), perceived loss of control was observed to lead to poor personal outcomes in schools, while studies by DiClemente, (1986) and Chapman, et al, (1990) found that a positive perception of control led to improved behaviour and successful performance.

Studies have also been conducted into internal and external LOC and age difference. In citing a total of sixteen previous studies, Lachman (1986) found that most of the previous studies fell into three categories: those who suggested that internal LOC decreased with age, those who suggested otherwise, and the third category of findings which suggested an equal status between both internal and external LOC in both adult and old age. The differences in study design, sampling, demography and measurement were given as possible explanation for the discrepancies in results (Lachman (1986; Cheng et al, 2013).

Lachman et al, (1990:38) further explored this by applying multidimensional measurement of both generalised and domain specific instruments and found that older groups were more external than internal compared to younger groups "for intelligence-specific chance control and health-specific powerful others control". Lachman stressed that the study further suggested that older individuals can retain their sense of internal control while accepting the importance of external sources of control (Lachman, 1986).

LOC has also been linked with individuals' experience with work and retirement, as it has been suggested that individuals tend to lean towards internal LOC during their active working life and exhibit more external orientation during their retirement years (Knoop (1989; Cheng et al, 2013). More recent studies which conducted literature reviewed into the exploration of LOC into several aspects of human affairs include academic works by Ponto (2004) and Papadopoulos (2009). Ponto (2004) highlighted a total of eight studies between 1980 and 2003 (Strickland & Haley, 1980; Knoop, 1989; Hall et al, 1997;

Carver, 1997; Wang et la, 1999; Leone & Burns, 2000; Santiago & Tarantino, 2002; and Judge et al, 2002), which examined the contribution of generalised LOC (Rotter, 1966) on human behaviour, especially in education settings. A more recent study into ethics education and Locus of Control stresses that a link exists between ethics education, 'leadership' and 'self-leadership' (Ogunyemi, 2013: 1). It was also suggested that "fostering or enhancing an internal locus of control is invaluable for people who are being prepared to be business leaders and hold managerial positions" (Ogunyemi, 2013: 17).

Majority of the identified studies which involved participants including teachers, students, and employees confirmed that internal and external LOC impacted upon or had some relevance on issues including "education and occupation", "age changes in working life and quality of life"; "interpersonal power and self-efficacy"; and other related issues (Ponto, 2004: 53). The latest review on available instruments on LOC by Cheng et al, (2013) asserts that more than 50 measuring instruments have emerged since Rotter's submission in 1966. The authors identified the Spheres of Control Scale by Paulhus and van Selst, (1990), Nowicki & Duke's, (1983) Adult Nowicki-Strickland Internal-External Control Scale (ANSIE), Duttweiler's, (1984) Internal Control Index; and Levenson's, (1981) Internality, Powerful Others and Chance Scales (IPCS) as the most popular tools in addition to Rotter's (1966) Internal-External Locus of Control Scale (RIES). It was also claimed that "These measures have undergone rigorous validation processes and have been shown to be applicable across a range of samples and contexts"(Cheng et al, 2013: 160), although a note of caution has been made in respect of the use of those measuring tools that were deemed not so popular.

3.2.4. LOC & Health

Various studies have explored the relationship between LOC and health in general, as well as specific areas of health seeking behaviours (Larson, (1989; Norman et al, 1998; Declerck et al, 2006; Poortinga, et al, 2008; Tigani, et al, 2011).

Earlier studies by Strickland, (1978), and Wallston & Wallston, (1981) on the link between LOC and health were based on applying the concept of Rotter's (1966) foundational model of internal and external LOC. Internals are those individuals who have the perception of control over their health while externals are individuals who believe that their health is not within their control (Wallston, 1992). It was also generally concluded in earlier studies that individuals located within the internal LOC spectrum are likely to participate in conducts and behaviours that will promote their health (Cheng et al, 2013; Tigani, et al, 2011). On the other hand, individuals who are of the external LOC orientation are likely to indulge more in behaviours which would not promote their health. Other authors including Seeman & Seeman, (1983) and Marshall, (1991) asserted that the differences in health behaviour profile between the individuals with internal LOC and those with external LOC will result in better health outcomes for the internals than the externals.

Studies have also explored the relationship between LOC and behavioural response to health promoting lifestyles, habits and encouragements. It has been found that individuals with internal LOC tend to subscribe to more health promoting lifestyles than those with external orientation, while individuals in the latter category are likely to be passive in this regard (Strickland, 1978; Mechanic & Cleary, 1980; Baranowski, 1984; Duffy, 1988; Rauckhorst, 1987; Cheng et al, 2013).

It was also found that the LOC orientation of individuals will also dictate the extent to which their health behaviour is influenced by the social environment and the influence of family and friends (Abella & Heslin, 1984). Strickland, (1977) suggests that individuals with internal LOC are less likely to submit to pressure from others to undertake poor health habits, as they are more likely to draw their own individual conclusion when confronted by opposing suggestions from external sources that they may find to be challenging their views and health related behaviours (Declerck et al, 2006).

In comparison, however, external LOC oriented persons may be more susceptible to the non-health promoting behaviour in their environment, either directly or indirectly, when exposed to similar situations (Declerck et al, 2006). External LOC oriented persons are also likely to be passive to health promoting behaviour, due to their tendency to place less value on their health as a result of perceived inability to control issues around their health (Abella & Heslin, 1984).

Weiss & Larsen, (1990) and Wallston, (1992) found that the value an individual place on their health would dictate their health behaviour (Norman et al, 1998). Tigani et al (2011), agrees that LOC is also indicated to influence health behaviours, as it characterizes the degree to which an individual takes personal responsibility in relation to the extent to which they perceive that their health outcomes was primarily due to fate, chance, or other groups' influence (powerful others, chance etc.), or the extent to which they believed that they had control over their health (Norman et al, 1998; Tigani et al, 2011).

One area that is seldom explored in relation to powerful others being in form of the medical and non-medical professionals and its impact on external LOC orientation was highlighted in a study by Norman et al, (1998). In the study that involved polling opinions of over 11,600 participants in Wales, in respect of Health Locus of Control, it confirmed findings of previous studies that internal LOC motivated positive health behaviour (Mechanic & Cleary, 1980; Seeman & Seeman, 1983; Rauckhorst, 1987; Duffy, 1988; Weiss & Larsen, 1990; Waller & Bates, 1992). It also confirmed the previous reports that a perception that one's health was controlled by fate and chance motivated poor health behaviour (Brown et al., 1983; Duffy, 1988; Muhlenkamp et al., 1985; Steptoe et al., 1994; Cheng et al, 2013; Declerck et al, 2006).

It was, however, discovered that individuals who have a strong belief in the role of powerful others are likely to perform lower levels of positive health behaviour (Norman et al, (1998; Declerck et al, 2006; Cheng et al, 2013). Norman et al (1998), had concluded earlier that "This suggests that, here, the powerful others HLC dimension reflects a belief in the ability of the medical profession to cure illness, and thereby protect health. Consequently, there may be less onus on the individual to engage in health-protecting behaviours" (Norman et al, 1998: 75). It, therefore, indicates a need for the health professions to promote health seeking behaviour by educating the populace on the need to take responsibility for one's health, promote internal LOC in individuals, which can encourage them to take active participation in the decision making on their health and embarking on healthy lifestyles to harness the benefits of the medical advice and procedures (Norman et al, 1998).

A study by Bennett et al (1997), into the HLOC (Health Locus of Control), value for health and frequency of smoking found that individuals who never smoked demonstrated a higher level of internal control and subscribed more to the influence of chance and powerful others. It was also discovered that the perceived influence of chance in the LOC played a significant role in the smoking behaviour of the study participants, just as those individuals who had stopped smoking ascribed higher value to their health than those who were smokers (Bennett et al, 1997). A more recent study by Tokuda et al, (2007) amongst adults in Japan found that people with higher internal HLOC used more complimentary alternative medicine and decreased professional control. It was suggested that the participants "consider alternative medicine to be less paternalistic, more empowering, and offering autonomy and control over their healthcare decision-making process" (Tokuda et al, 2007: 648).

3.2.5. LOC & General Health – Measurement scales

Some research into the internal and external (I-E) LOC measures specific to health include that of Kirscht (1972), which focused on some predictive value of scale for health-related behaviour to determine a perception of control of health; and Wallston et al. (1976), which was based on an 11 item scale to predict health-related behaviour. The two scales were found to have considered health in terms of physical wellbeing, while Wallston et al (1976) scale was found to "showed discriminant validity when contrasted with Rotter's I-E Scale" (Wood & Letak, 1982: 85).

Others include multidimensional health LOC measures developed in recognition that LOC was not one-dimensional but multidimensional. These scales by (Wallston, Wallston & Devellis,

(1978); Lau & Ware, (1981), and Lau, 1982), not only assessed LOC on health, but provided instruments that measure the extent to which health LOC can be credited to the influence of powerful others and chance. Wood & Letak (1982: 85) found that the scales were characteristically "multidimensional" and that the factors "that most frequently have emerged have included:

- Perceptions that luck or fate controls events;
- Beliefs that one can influence political or social systems; and
- Perceived self-control"

A study was conducted by Marshall et al (1990), to evaluate the LOC measuring instruments developed by Wallston et al (1978), and Lau (1982), in order to measure the extent to which the two instruments could be merged for use, along with "internal consistency, reliability, factor structure, and construct validity" (Marshall et al (1990: 188). The study found that both multidimensional instruments were not highly convergent because they found that, "internal consistency reliability" of the Lau (1982) LOC scales were poorer than the Wallston et al, (1978) instruments (Marshall et al, 1990: 182).

Further studies into measuring health LOC was based on the premise that four identified health behaviours play significant role in health outcomes. These behaviours were categorised into two parts – those behaviours that promote health and those that exert limitation on health. The health promoting behaviours include exercise and healthy eating habits, while health-limiting behaviours include smoking and excessive alcohol consumption (Amler& Eddings, 1987; Norman et al, 1998).

Furthermore, it was observed that the main limitation of Multidimensional LOC (MHLC) scale lies in its measurement of behaviours which are based on their beliefs in general (generalised beliefs), which in turn depends on the limited knowledge of individuals (Norman et al, 1998). This indicates an individual's perception of control will depend on their level of knowledge, which, in turn, dictates their behaviour. It is, therefore, deemed necessary to measure behaviours not on generalised expectancies but on specific domains, as the knowledge of the domains impact on expectancies, and consequently on the behaviours (Norman et al, 1998).

Research in this area have resulted in development of LOC measuring scales for domain specific areas, which have been suggested to offer predictive behaviour pattern than generalised expectancies (Lefcourt, 1991; Norman et al, 1998). Some of these include measuring scales for LOC on the relationship between LOC and smoking by Georgiou & Bradley, (1992), and Bennett et al, (1997); LOC and exercise (Burk & Kimiecik, 1994), AIDS-risk behaviour (Kelley et al, 1990), and LOC and weight loss (Saltzer, 1982). Others include LOC and the use of alcohol (Donovan & O'Leary, 1978), Health LOC and the use of conventional and alternative health care (Tokuda et al, 2007).

A more recent report by Halpert and Hill, (2011) found that the Multidimensional Health Locus of Control (MHLOC) scale have been found to be generally more reliable and has been popular in health promotion programs. The scale has also been applied in studies investigating ageing and LOC (Bailis et al, 2010); LOC and behaviour concerning nutrition (Chen et al, 2010); LOC and cancer in individuals aged 60 and over (Knappe & Pinquart, 2009); and LOC in persons experiencing lower back pain (Sengul et al, 2010). However, there were no reports of validity or measurement of reliability included in the reports.

3.2.6. LOC & Mental Health

As indicated at the start of this chapter, this review also conducted searches into databases and professional journals to identify studies into the specific relevance of LOC to mental health. Most of the studies found were, however, dominated by general health topics rather than specifically mental health focus. In addition, most of the studies were not only dated, as they were conducted about twenty years ago, they were also based in western countries including the United States of America, Australia, and the United Kingdom (Cheng et al, 2013).

It was also found that specific focus in relation to particular mental health diagnosis (such as schizophrenia and Bipolar disorders) and their link with LOC has not been intensively explored, except for the link of LOC with other psychological health conditions such as depression and anxiety which have been attracting more intensive attention, including design of tools to measure depression and anxiety (Cheng et al, (2013).

The attributes of sense of well-being, quality of life, and psychological well-being have been rated to be closely determined by LOC orientation, and impact on general health and wellbeing (Poortinga, et al, 2008). Earlier studies by Thompson (1981) indicated that a perception of control over one's circumstances enables one to cope more with stressful conditions. Just as stressful situations can be coped with by a perception of control (Taylor, Lichtman, & Wood, 1984), a perception of a loss of control will often lead to poor health outcomes for the person. This was indicated in the studies about hospital patients (Taylor, 1979) and elderly nursing homes (Slivinske & Fitch, 1987).

LOC has also been found to play active role in mental health, as it has been advanced that there is a positive correlation between LOC and aspects of mental health (Declerck et al, 2006; Cheng et al, 2013). It has also been suggested that LOC is a stronger predictor of subjective well-being and happiness than conscientiousness, emotional stability, or extraversion alone (Declerck et al, 2006). Larson, (1989) suggests that a perception of having control over one's life has a positive correlation with improved physical and emotional health.

Studies that have explored the link between LOC and mental health have mostly focused on its link with depression. They include Benassi, et al (1988); Holder & Levi, (1988); Wang, Wang, & Zhang, (1992); Akande & Lester, (1994); and Tobin & Raymundo, (2010). All these studies found a positive correlation between depression and LOC, with additional information from the meta analytic review studies by Benassi, et al (1988) which confirmed a higher link between external LOC and depression (Cheng et al, 2013). The latest meta-analysis conducted by Cheng et al, (2013) also supported this view with additional findings that LOC is positively correlated with anxiety.

Earlier studies into mental health related LOC also found a positive correlation between life stresses, depression and anxiety on one hand and external locus of control on the other (Johnson & Sarason, 1978). A study was also conducted by Birchwood et al, (1993) which undertook a comparison of the LOC and depression profile of individuals with psychotic illness. It was found that people with more chronic forms of psychosis tend to have a higher level of external LOC than those who experience less chronic levels of psychosis.

Holmberg & Kane (1999) also conducted a study in which higher external scores were reported by participants with schizophrenia, which also indicated that these client groups tend to have a higher level of external health LOC compared with the general population. Judge et al, (2002) also found that in comparison with other members of the public, the experience of personality disorders leads to external LOC in the sufferers.

A more recent study by Buhagiar, et al, (2011) at an out-patient adult mental health service in London (UK) conducted a cross-sectional comparison to determine general health LOC between the clients with psychotic and non-psychotic mental illness. It was found that the patients with psychotic diagnosis demonstrated greater level of external LOC compared to the non-psychotic patients. This was exhibited more in "powerful others" such as family members, and "chance". This confirms findings from previous studies, (Johnson &Sarason, 1978; Birchwood et al, 1993; Holmberg & Kane, 1999), although those studies involved non-psychotic populations.

3.2.6.1. Summary-LOC & Mental Health

This review indicates that most of the studies have found a positive correlation between external LOC and mental illness experience (Wood & Letak, 1982; Johnson & Sarason, 1978; Birchwood et al, 1993; Holmberg & Kane, 1999; Judge et al., 2002; Buhagiar, Parsonage and Osborn, 2011). This suggests that the varying degrees and types of mental illness including psychotic and non-psychotic illness experiences tend to make the individuals more prone to becoming external in their LOC. It has also been found that the perception of groups from BME populations regarding the aetiology of the mental illness they experienced has a relationship to their LOC (McCabe & Priebe, 2004).

3.2.7. LOC, Mental Health & Culture in the United Kingdom

In relation to the relationship between culture and LOC of BME population, it was also found that a few United Kingdom based studies have explored culture and LOC from the experiences of the BME peoples with mental health and MHS. Papadopoulos' (2009) study was the only recent study found to have explored LOC in individualism and collectivism in the context of stigma. The study was based on study participants in the United Kingdom of white-English, American, Greek/Greek Cypriot, and Chinese groups. No other study was found to have investigated the concept of individualism and collectivism in LOC as it relates to mental health in BME populations that included other Asian, African and Caribbean peoples.

The closest study to this concept was by McCabe and Priebe (2004). This was a study involving schizophrenia patients from four cultural backgrounds (UK Whites and Bangladeshis, African Caribbeans and West Africans) which explored LOC in the contexts of explanatory model, clinical and mental characteristics in their experience of schizophrenia. It was found that the study participants' belief regarding the aetiology of their illness had a bearing on their LOC as well as the profile of their satisfaction with the treatment they received. It also indicated that participant's experience of using mental health services had a positive correlation with what they believed about their illness (McCabe and Priebe (2004). This study was, however, more focused on explanatory models for aetiology of mental illness rather than influence of culture on LOC orientation, its relationship to and experiences of mental health services.

3.2.8. The Applicability of Locus of Control for Black & Minority Ethnic (BME) Mental Health

> *"...when it comes to the correlations between locus of control and aspects of psychological health, the locus control is a stronger predictor of subjective well-being and happiness...."* (Declerck et al, 2006: 147)

As indicated above by Declerck et al (2006), LOC has been found to play an important role in aspects of psychological health (including individual wellbeing, happiness and life satisfaction) as well as various dimensions of personality (Judge et al., 2004, Declerck et al, 2006; Cheng et al, 2013). It is also reported to be not only a product of social learning, but has a bearing on biological foundation and connotations, including its relationship with the effect of neurotransmitters such as dopamine levels in the human brain, which, in turn, impact on the human capacity to regulate self and direct one's behaviours (Declerck et al, 2006).

Declerck et al (2006: 146) also found that various lines of thought and many longitudinal and cross-cultural studies indicated that LOC is based within what has been termed "the Big 5" dimensions of personality (Declerck et al, 2006: 146). These include Emotional stability, Conscientiousness, Agreeableness, Openness and Extraversion (Declerck et al, (2006:146). LOC is, therefore, considered a great instrument for the prediction of psychological health and evaluation of subjective wellbeing, happiness, and satisfaction (Kirkcaldy, Shephard, & Funham, 2002; Declerck et al, 2002).

LOC has also been highlighted to raise issues that explain the perception of control from different cultural perspectives (Triandis & Suh, 2002; Triandis, 1995b; Marcus & Kitayama, 1999; Cheng et al., 2013). It has also identified differences that exist between the approach of individualist societies (a characteristic of the mainstream population) to control, and the approach of the collectivist societies, which the Black and Minority Ethnic (BME) community belongs (Cheng et al, 2013).

LOC, therefore, offers an opportunity to explore the possibility or likelihood that the BME perception of control as well as the identified differences between the BME community's perception and that of the mainstream population may have some bearing with the state of dissatisfaction of the BME community with services (Cheng et al, 2013). It also presents a prospect to explore the likelihood that LOC can be considered to be a factor in, as well as present some explanation for the challenges stipulated above in the experiences of the BME clients, their carers and family members with mental health services (Cheng et al, 2013). This also indicates that LOC could present a greater understanding for the identified experience of crisis entry pathway, overrepresentation, and coercive practices, observed disparities in care and outcomes and overall dissatisfaction of BME groups with MHS (Cheng et al, 2013).

This forms the basis for the use of LOC as an approach to address the knowledge gap in this area and a logical approach to take advantage of the opportunity it presents to unearth the possible cultural foundational basis for the identified BME mental health challenges. This is with the ultimate view to proffering solutions for the current situation and the challenges it presents.

Although it is not part of the conceptual framework for this study, it has been stressed that the evolution of cultural psychiatry in Great Britain have led to a greater focus on the challenges relating to the experience of ethnic minorities (Littlewood, 1992). Concerns were related to suspected misdiagnosis of BME and immigrant groups (Littlewood, 1992), higher rates of schizophrenia diagnosis in Black patients compared to the White population, and proportionately higher rates of coercive practices such as detention being experienced by ethnic minorities (Dunn & Fahy, 1990; Bebbington et al., 1994; Cole et al, 1995; Bhui et al, 2014). This has culminated in more suggestions by cultural psychiatrists that the mental health problems of ethnic minorities be accorded more attention and resources (Bains, 2005). However, it has also been asserted that future research can be successful by eliminating the concept of cultural psychiatry as a separate discipline and turning "all mental health research into the study of cultures in society, within which mental health care can be positioned" (Bhui & Singh, 2004: 127).

The exploration of LOC as a conceptual framework was also a logical preference for the researcher, as it was intended to utilise it as a foundation towards addressing the issues. This is also in view of the findings that indicated that internal and external LOC has correlation with human behaviour in health and other contexts, including but not limited to regulation of self and emotion directed coping styles (Hess & Vossel, 2001; Huizink, et al, 2002); reasoning functions and social cognition (Declerck et al, 2006); and in the psychopathology of schizophrenia (Chadwick, 2001; Declerck et al, 2006).

4| Power, Care, Control and Coercion

4.1. Introduction

This section explores the concepts of Power, Care, Control, and Coercion in the context of mental health and social care, including their theoretical basis. It discusses the relationship between these concepts and their influence on the experiences of clients in mental health and social care. It suggests that the four concepts are inextricably linked and need to be considered in the narratives relating to the overall experiences of mental health clients, their family members, and carers. It also indicates that these concepts need to be considered from the domain of the role played by the culture and ethnicity of groups from the BME community, particularly A & C communities in their LOC and in their overall experience with mental health services.

4.2. Power in Mental Health Services

> *Power refers to the ability to have one's will carried out despite the resistance of others*
>
> (Barkhan, 2012: 558)

This section reviews the theoretical basis around power and its application to health and social care, with focus on mental health services. It explores the various schools of thought on the concept including pre and post-modernist approaches, and theories. By focusing on knowledge and agency as inherent basis of power in mental health and social care, it concludes with the findings that health and social care need to be constantly aware and keep cognisance of the intricacies of power in building relationships and the overall engagement of mental health service professionals with the mental health service clients, their careers, and family members.

4.2.1. Theories on Power

Several theories exist on power, which have evolved over time. The basic concept of power refers to one party being able to exert control over another party (Hui & Stickley, 2007; Barry, 2013). This suggests that there is a sense of dominance of groups over others (Hui & Stickley, 2007). This includes the concept of power being a commodity that is quantifiable, and transferable from one group to another. Power is also exerted by coercion, where someone is made to "agree" to do things they would not normally willingly subscribe to (Hui & Stickley, 2007).

Power has also been described as a concept that is fundamentally contested, like democracy, justice and equality (Barry, 2013). It has also been asserted that power is also inherently political, with the existence of interdependency between power and politics (Barry, 2013). This indicates that power could almost be interchangeably applied in relation to politics, as it has been asserted that "Theoretical perspectives on power are, to a large extent, theoretical perspective on politics itself. That is, definitions of power are constitutive of what we mean by politics and the political" (Barry, 2013: 4). This concept also defines power based on three theories- Elitist, Pluralist and Marxist (Barry, 2013). Pluralism focuses on how power is distributed, with insider groups being more powerful than outsider groups (Barry, 2013). Elitism focuses on how power is concentrated, with a small class of people holding power and decision making over the larger population; while Marxism is interested in the conflict between classes of power and economic power by producing and protecting capitalism towards regulating social and political stability (Barry, 2013;Barkhan, 2012). Gender theory of power states that power is concentrated in the hands of men in the society who operates as a group, making the women in the society to be the dominated group, including leadership positions (Schuh et al, 2014).

Other concepts of power include the multidimensional notion which terms power as a construct originated from innately social, cultural and institutional sources, which, in turn, dictates specific patterns of behaviour within the society (Lukes, 1994). It is also asserted that this construct means that power is highly concentrated in the hands of the majority population in the society which tend to exert its cultural dominance, ideas and intent/agenda on the rest of the population (Hugman, 1991). This leads to inequality in the society and the dominance of the minority (Barry, 2013).

The post-modernist approach to power relies on the importance of knowledge as the driving force and basis of power in the society. This view is championed by Foucault's (1980) assertion of knowledge and power being "inseparable" entities, as knowledge, communication and learning promotes power. It has also been asserted that value placed upon professional knowledge marginalizes local knowledge, or 'subjugated knowledge' (Jupp, 2005:3). In the same vein communication and knowledge are seen by the post-modernists as fundamental in understanding power within society" (Jupp, 2005: 1).

Foucault suggests that power can be exploited in several ways, by language, action or repetition (Foucault, 2001). As a result, diverse roles and responsibilities become official within society, which then becomes the social norm and so-called socially constructed truths that develop within societies (Foucault, 2001). Foucault also highlights the importance played by so called "professional knowledge" or "professional discourse" which becomes the "dominant truth" (Pease, 2002: 141), and in turn tend to promote the marginalisation of other knowledge. This is because those who have gained power with this dominant discourse could then fashion their own version of history and consequential 'truths', that prevent due knowledge and consideration of other equally significant historical events that may have less power. This is referred to as 'discursive formations' (Sarup, 1993; Foucault, 2001). The consequence of this lies in the likelihood that discrimination is promoted, and minority views become subjugated in the society (Sarup, 1993; Foucault, 2001).

Foucault also discusses the concept of power from a disciplinary domain, describing it as disciplinary power (Foucault, 1977), which is found in all aspects of the society, and as necessary for management of people. He highlighted some of these discipline power as being dominant and operative in prisons (Foucault, 1977), in households, for example, patriarchal family dynamics (Foucault 1985, 1986), and asylums (Foucault, 2006). The disciplinary connotations were also highlighted as containing both necessary enabling and restricting elements (Foucault 1978). It was also observed that disciplinary power is diffused (i.e., it cannot be ascribed to one or several persons) (Foucault, 1977; Broer, et al, 2012), and utilises numerous methods to manage people (Broer, et al, 2012).

The method applied in ruling people can involve the use of language and planned practices, which can be either discursive or non-discursive. It has also been observed that from a Foucauldian viewpoint, all these techniques rely upon esoteric knowledge practices. Every form of knowledge is also set as a rule, which includes norms that are presumed to be for 'normal' behaviour and those which are considered for behaviours that are considered 'deviant' (that is unexpected in the society) (Foucault 2010). Foucault, (2010) also asserts that as such knowledge has regulated normalised behaviour in the society, it tends to order reality. Consequently, knowledge itself becomes an intervention tool just as it suggests how to further impact on the society. Foucault referred to this reciprocal constitution between forms of knowledge and power techniques as 'governmentality' (Lemke 2001; Foucault 2010).

4.2.2 Implications of Power for Mental Health Service Provision and Experience

Professional knowledge and its relationship to power also plays a role in the imbalance of power between the mental health practitioner who is perceived to have professional knowledge, on the one hand and the mental health clients on the other; and impacts on the perception, response to and ultimate recovery for the latter (Morrow & Weisser, 2012).

The health professionals are, therefore, not only seen as a representative of the Mental Health Services (MHS) in the provision of care, they are also seen as the presence and appearance of those in possession of the power to take decisions that impact on the lives of the clients (Jupp, 2005).

The power held by the service provider which is embedded in the provisions of the MHA (1983, 2007; DoH, 2015), allows for the mental health professionals working for the respective health trusts, and ultimately the State, to apply the powers in the Act. The Act has been likened to be in the same status with the provisions of the counter terrorism act 1974 (Prevention of Terrorism Act 1974 and the National Assistance Act 1948) in its statutory provision of detaining persons and depriving them of their liberty without adhering to the provisions of the law that requires people to appear before a judicial body (Sullivan, 1998). However, this viewpoint appears to be countered by the provision in the MHA whereby patients have a right to appeal to the hospital managers as well as have their case referred to mental health Tribunals (Brown, 2016; Barber et al, 2012).

Another issue around power lies in the provision that the Mental Health Trust is given the legal powers under the Act to detain and treat people deemed to be mentally ill as inpatients (Brown, 2016). However, this provision is also moderated by the provision of the MHA which allows for three sets of professionals including the individual's General Practitioner (GP), a Responsible Clinician (RC), and an Approved Mental Health Practitioner (AMHP) (Brown, 2016). The MHA also allows the Trust to monitor and recall people who have mental illness from the community for readmission into hospitals by the imposition of Community Treatment Orders (CTOs), (Brown, 2016). This is also, in turn, regulated by a provision that such decisions must be guided by a multidisciplinary team of professionals (Maden & Spencer-Lane, 2010; Jones, 2011; Brown, 2016; Barber et al, 2012).

The provision of the Section 136 of the MHA also gives the power to the police to detain and take people found in a public place believed to be suffering from mental disorder, to a place of safety, a hospital, and other places, where they are assessed under the Act, and referred for psychiatric assessment and admission if needed (DoH, 2015; Brown, 2016). This highlights the existence of the potential of the police also becoming perceived as agents of coercion emanating from the power given the police under the Act to detain. The police can, therefore, be agents of the state who are authorised to deny someone their liberty on the suspicion of the existence of mental illness and the perceived need for such a person to be taken to a place of safety for assessment. However, the Act provides that such power can only be exercised where there is a perceived risk to the safety of the individual and/or other members of the public, and the legal criteria for such detention must be met (Jones, 2011).

Such deprivation of liberty can also be seen as a tool of coercion and control due to the exercise of power by the police under the Act, which may not be necessary at the time, as the decision of the police team to detain such a person could be perceived as subjective. This has been played out in reality where reports have indicated that some cases involving people taken and detained in "places of safety" by the police under the suspicion that they were suffering from mental illness whilst utilising the provision of section 136 of the MHA have resulted in the persons being deemed as having no mental illness post assessment by health professionals, and had resulted in them being allowed to go home and carry on with their lives (CQC, 2013).

However, such deprivation of liberty is waived because there is no recourse against the police for such unfair detention by utilising the provisions of the MHA, for the period it had taken before the member of the public released, and the consequent sense of anger, fear, suspicion and potential mistrust of the MHA and the police who are seen as agents of coercion, force and deprivation of freedom. With respect to the places of safety in hospitals, a recent Care Quality Commission report on the statistics of such detention in England resulting in nil admission states that:

> *"Only 17 % of recorded uses of hospital-based places of safety under section 136 resulted in further detention, following assessment by mental health professionals"* (CQC, 2013: 3).

This highlights the potential impact of actual deprivation of liberty on the response of people who have experienced mental illness and have been subjected to such treatment, even if their detention experience had resulted in being sectioned for treatment.

Another example of the provisions of the Act is the power given to the police to enter a premise under Section 135, to search for and remove a 'patient'. However, the Act requires that there needs to be evidence that the person is suffering from mental disorder, may be experiencing ill treatment, neglected, kept otherwise than under proper control or unable to care for themselves in the given area (Brown, 2016).

The Act provides that an AMHP obtains a warrant from a magistrates' court to enter clients' premises to assess their needs under the company of the police (Brown, 2016). There is also a limitation as to how long such individuals can be detained, as they can be removed to a place of safety for up to 72 hours (Maden & Spencer-Lane, 2010; Jones, 2011). This indicates that the Act also makes provision to ensure that no one is deprived of their liberty without genuine reasons for the safety of themselves and other members of the public and the operation of appropriate safeguards (Brown, 2016). It also indicates that the overarching principles of the Act include least restrictive option, maximising independence, empowerment and involvement, respect and dignity, and purpose and effectiveness (Barber et al, 2012; DoH, 2015).

The impact of the detentions on the potential of the response of the clients to interventions that are aimed to support, lead to or aid their recovery is also highlighted. It has been suggested that

> *"central to any discussion about recovery must be recognition of the profound discrimination faced by people who have been psychiatrized, and the connections between recovery and the social and structural barriers that shape, facilitate or impede recovery"* (Morrow & Weisser, 2012: 28).

This indicates that in order to impact positively on the recovery of their clients, the mental health practitioners need to be aware of their role as agents of the mental health services (MHS), the imbalance of power between themselves, and the clients and within the structure of the health services including the coercive actions the system had taken in the journey of the mental health clients. This may include the need to be aware of what has been termed *"internalized oppression"* (Jupp, 2005:8), which is rooted in powerlessness that may be experienced by the clients in the relationship dichotomy (Jupp, 2005).

This is, however, tempered by the sources of succour available to the clients in the overarching guiding principles and criteria for detentions in the MHA (Barber et al, 2012; DoH, 2015) expected to be adhered to by the respective Mental Health Trusts.

The provisions in the Equality Act (2010), (Barber et al, 2012) are also aimed at addressing discrimination on account of disability that arises from some mental health conditions (Mind, 2017). The provision of the Code of Practice (Barber et al, 2012) also guides the application of the MHA, and is monitored through inspections by the CQC (Barber et al, 2012; CQC, 2016). This is in addition to the provision that the Trusts must always use the least restrictive option, which, in turn, would make detention to be a last resort action (CQC, 2013). The clients also have the right to appeal their detention through the First Tier Tribunal and Hospital Managers (the Board), as well as a right to Independent Mental Health Advocates, IMHA (CQC, 2013).

The existence of such provisions can only be of effect if the clients are made aware of their rights under the MHA (1983, 2007) and how they can access such support. This has been addressed as it is a legal requirement that the CQC inspect Trusts for compliance in this area, thereby providing that hospital managers adhere to the provision (Brown, 2016). The rights of clients as indicated in the MHA (2007) are also expected to be communicated to them by the mental health professionals, especially at such periods of their lives that they are most vulnerable (Barber et al, 2012; Brown, 2016).

On the other hand, it has been asserted that power also exists in the hands of the clients, including the power to demand independence as well as expression of their opinion regarding the care they receive in the community (Dalley, 1994). However, it has been found that the exercise of these powers is limited by the fact that the clients "equate caring with control", and "that the way in which disability is socially constructed forces those with impairments into the control of informal carers or official service providers" (Dalley, 1994:425). This includes availing themselves of the provision of after discharge care as embedded in section 117 of the MHA, (Golightley, 2014) as well as the Care Planning Approach (CPA) (Brown, 2016). This section of the Act aims to enable clients to return to the community and minimise re-hospitalisation.

It also makes it the duty of services and local governments to provide aftercare services to those who have been detained for treatment under section 3 of the Act, as well as support services which may include employment, housing, occupation, and training (DoH, 2015; CQC, 2014). In addition, two important laws relating to human rights also constitute important safeguards against abuse of the rights of mental health clients. These are the Human Rights Act 1998, (Brown, 2016), which came into effect in the year 2000, and the European Convention on Human Rights (ECHR) (Brown, 2016). Articles 3 and 5 of the Human Rights Act (1998) covers issues including torture, inhuman or degrading treatment or punishment; right to liberty and security of persons (Barber et al, 2012; Brown, 2016). The provisions of the MHA (2007), its Code of Practice and the amendments made to the Mental Capacity Act (Brown, 2016), are also combined with the Deprivation of Liberty Safeguards (DoLS) which covers aspects of control within the mental health settings to protect the rights of the clients (Brown, 2016). Brown (2016) surmised that three main features have been identified as factors in determining DoLS. They include "the objective component of confinement in a particular restricted place for a not negligible length of time; and the subjective component of a lack of valid consent; and the attribution of responsibility to the state" (Brown, 2016: 148).

All public authorities, including the Approved Mental Health Practitioners (AMHPs), approved clinicians, doctors, psychiatrists, and institutions including the Care Quality Commission, the courts, tribunals, the NHS and local authorities are expected to defer to the ECHR rights, unless they are prevented by statue (Brown, 2016). Indeed, the European Court has been known to have ruled against services in respect of clients being subject to breaches of the Human Rights Act (Brown, 2016). This includes the Bournwood case (2004), where breaches of Articles 5.1 and 5.4 relating to deprivation of liberty have been decided by the Court (Barber et al, 2012; Brown, 2016). This indicates that mental health clients can exercise their rights to prevent controls that they consider a breach of their human rights.

Additional safeguards are also provided in sections 57 and 58 of the MHA (2007), whereby Second Opinion Appointed Doctors (SOADs) can be appointed by the Care Quality Commission (CQC) in England (and Healthcare Inspectorate Wales, for clients in Wales) to review treatments proposed by Approved Clinicians (AC), when it is deemed required (Brown, 2016). This requires the SOADs to provide an independent report on their opinion as to whether a treatment proposed by the AC should go ahead or be withheld on the grounds of 'serious harm' (Brown, 2016: 132). This indicates that the clients' rights can be protected by having his needs, views and opinions considered through a review by an SOAD, as covered by section 25.60, 25.61 and 25.62 of the MHA (2007). (Brown, 2016)

In addition to the above-mentioned safeguards, professional power of services and other public authorities have been challenged by service user movements and in mental and other health settings (Kalathil, 2009; Seebohm et al, 2013). They can also form client's groups which can act as agents of change by seeking to involve clients in the overall provision of the services they receive (Baldwin & Sadd, 2006; Brown, 2016). An example of this is found in the involvement of clients as "allies" in the running of social work education courses (Baldwin & Sadd, 2006). The formation of active clients' pressure groups (also known as service user movements) (Baldwin & Sadd, 2006) were galvanised in the voluntary sector and aimed at partnering with the mainstream services in order to provide more support to service users in partnership with statutory agencies (Campbell et al, 2004; NHS, 2016). However, such partnerships between BME voluntary organisations and statutory services have been seen to have contributed to marginalisation of the BME populations, due to non-involvement of these groups in active decision making and the challenges of funding (Campbell, 2004). Such marginalisation has also been characterised by insecurity in funding and short-term contracts; these, in turn, has limited their ability to harness opportunities to support the communities (Campbell, 2004; Fernando & Keating, 2009; Keating, 2016).

4.3. Care in Mental Health

> *"In the relationship between the carer and the cared-for, there is a continual tension on the part of the cared-for between wanting and appreciating care and resenting it"* (Lupton, 1997, p.105).

4.3.1. Care- Origin, Meaning and Paradox

The development of caring has emerged as a concept of importance in nursing since the 1950s and following Nightingale's (1859) assertion that the greatest imperative work in nursing is caring (Meng, et al, 2011). Caring has, therefore, been the heart of the nursing vocation (Leininger 1984a; Brilowski & Wendler 2005; Meng, et al, 2011). Various schools of thought on caring has included subjecting the concept to theories including systems of values of human caring suggested by Watson (1979; 2008) including hope, sensitivity, trust, faith and relationship. It also includes practicing loving-kindness and calmness, honouring, being genuinely present, enabling and other attributes (Watson (1979; 2008). Caring also has the dual meaning of 'caring for someone' and 'caring about someone' (Thomas 1993: 649).

Theories on the motivation behind people caring also exists over disciplines, including, economic, instinctiveness and biological makeup; a form of barter based on rituals; while others insist that caring is motivated by commitment, religion and power; and societal expectations have been adduced for caring from the sociological perspectives (Wiseman, 1997).

The dual meaning and the tendency of mutual exclusivity of the terms "caring for" and "caring about" therefore indicates the need to explore their implications for health care in general and mental health (Fox 1995; Graham, 1983; Lynch, 1989; Wiseman 1997). Caring for indicates actions taken to tend for someone while the idea of caring about another person emanates from the emotional state of what has been termed as "feeling" for another person (Wiseman 1977). The difference in these two terms lies in the fact that one could tend for someone without having any feeling or "care" about them. This means that there is propensity for one to not be interested in someone's wellbeing whilst treating them, and take care of someone whilst being completely devoid of any emotional attachment towards the wellbeing of that person, although Wiseman suggests that "the latter will motivate the former" (Wiseman 1977: 44).

Caring has also been explored from a feminist and historical perspective (Dalley, 1996), in which it has been posited that the practice of care in the community has placed people with experience of disability, the aged as well as female carers at a disadvantage. It was articulated that this situation was due to flawed assumptions about what constitutes an ideal model of family life. A contrast between what was termed an "individualist" or "familist" orientation to caring, which historically assigns the caring role to the female, to a "collectivist" approach has been raised (Dalley, 1996). It was recommended that a more "collectivist" approach should be taken to caring, whereby roles are equally assigned to both male and female members, rather than suppressing the female gender, as well as the need to promote equality in gender, race and social class (Dalley, 1996: 107).

In Fox's (1995) exploration of what he referred to as what "postmodernism and poststructuralism perspective bring to an understanding of care", he suggests that "care is paradoxical" (Fox, 1995: 108). This irony lies in the fact that caring has been professionalised which in turn has created the need for caring to be a subject of scrutiny and monitoring. This consequently created the need for control in the profession. The professionalization (the creation of a discipline) of caring which has resulted in scrutiny and monitoring has also been described as a form of control, which in turn "supplies the authority for profession care' (Fox, 1995:108). Gardner (1992) asserts that the two fold contrasts in care lie in the fact that caring is based on relationships that rate the importance of being helpful, giving, and showing concern to the other person on the one hand, whilst on the other hand the practices of caring are based on a body of knowledge, professionalism and codes of practices.

This lends credence to the position that this creation of discipline (Fox, 1995), acts as a source of power and legitimacy to the people who practice care, and thus creates what has been termed by Foucault (1978) as 'docile bodies' of the people who are in receipt of care (Fox, 1995:108). Discipline has been described as a term that "means both a set of practices by which individuals become subjects of power, and secondly a professional or academic grouping" (Fox 1995: 111). Caring is not only an act that is necessary for certain conveyed need of another person, but also an activity that health practitioners can claim that what they are conducting in their caring profession is not only necessary but are also legitimate and valuable to the recipients of their care.

By the creation of the caring discipline with authority, it also creates the notion of the carer and the cared-for, which makes the cared-for the subject of the carer (Hugman, 1991). This creation of discipline based on knowledge and codified practices are inextricably linked with power and authority, as Foucault (1980), submits that power is complexly connected with knowledge. It suggests that this knowledge that has stemmed from concepts of care, therefore, gives more weight to power and control than with values of love, trust and giving which is supposed to be the overriding aim of care as a concept in the first instance (Fox, 1995; Hugman, 1991). This would suggest that the position of professionalism in care has the tendency to make one consider it as only a profession rather than having a genuine sense of caring about the person one is caring for in the health setting. This has been referred to by Fox (1995: 114) as "a technology of surveillance which, as a consequence of the professionalization of caring, constitutes the vigil".

4.3.2. Implications of the Care Paradox in Mental Health

It has been asserted that mental health theory and practice evolved "driven principally by tensions between different perspectives regarding the causes of mental health problems and how best to respond to these and the people affected by them. There is particular debate regarding whether this should be on a voluntary or involuntary basis for the benefit of the individual patient or the wider community" (Hardy, 2015: 53). In addition, as the MHA is also considered a response to this observed debate regarding voluntary and involuntary treatment by making specific provisions by which the professional is supposed to provide 'care' to the clients. These present some implications; one of which may operate in the mental health setting whereby the mental health professional could be considered by the patient to be less interested in the wellbeing of their patients as long as they have observed the provisions of the profession as it relates to adhering to the professionalism and the control that accompanies and governs the profession.

It would also suggest that a social worker or mental health nurse could decide to relate to the patients only on a professional basis only if he/she is acting within the coercive provisions of the MHA (2007), without any sense or consideration for the opinions, wellbeing or feeling of the mental health patient. This contrasts heavily with the standpoint that caring refers to a feeling of sense of kindness, attention, concern and commitment for people's wellbeing amongst other attributes (Roach, 1987; Brilowski & Wendler, 2005; Watson, 1979, 2008). This is even more poignant in view of the fact that in this case the overriding motive for caring 'for' someone in the mental health setting could be seen as emanating from an obligatory responsibility as the health professional being the carer in this case is paid for the services rendered to the patient, rather than a feeling of compassion to care for the mental health clients.

4.3.3. Control in Mental Health Services, Tension with Care?

The preceding section on care, its paradox as well as the implications in mental health settings in turn highlights the concept of control, its relationship with care, and the tension that arises there from. It has been submitted that control has been identified as an obvious goal of care (Glasser & Bridgeman, 1999), while although it may not be intended, control invariably becomes a consequence of care provision of care (Schneider, 2010). The role of social work in relation to the care-control tension has also been highlighted in the contexts of the necessity to take a social approach to mental health. It has been asserted that "mental health social work emerged in response to a perceived need within the mental health system for a less coercive and more socially oriented counterpoint to the dominance of medical psychiatry and asylums" (Hardy, 2015: 52). In further reference to the negative consequence of the authority and power created for the care practitioners from the knowledge-based discipline (Fox, 1995), it has been highlighted that this creates a feeling of the need to comply and reciprocate to the care-giver from the care receiver's point of view. This further creates a feeling of a lack of control and disempowerment for the care receiver (Schneider, 2010).

The tension between care and control is also played out from the provisions of the MHA (1983, 2007) on the one hand and the perspectives of the service providers, their agents and the clients on the other (Sullivan, 1998; CQC, 2013). In a bid to protect the members of the public as well as the rights of individuals, the MHA is a legal tool that governs the care and treatment of individuals who are subject to compulsory intervention, including the settings and processes under which individuals could be detained and treated for mental illness (Sullivan, 1998; CQC, 2013). For example, the Act provides guidelines for 'holding powers' which can be applied against informal patients (those who have not been 'sectioned' and could decide to exercise their rights to self-discharge) in inpatient mental health settings. A further demonstration of the interplay of the care and control tension, in which control tend to be more accentuated for such informal patients can be said to be demonstrated in a 2013 CQC report. This report found that section 5(2) of the Act, which permits doctors to direct that a patient be held for up to 72 hours on the grounds that the doctor needed that time to decide that an application should be made for further detention of such patients, was used most frequently in 2012 and 2013 (CQC, 2013).

It was also reported that nurses were also authorised by section 5(4) of the Act to detain patients for up to six hours where a doctor is not immediately available to apply section 5(2), where it is deemed necessary to "prevent an informal inpatient from leaving hospital" (CQC, 2013: 15), until a doctor is available. This indicates that although the mental health services were deemed to be providing care to the patient, the latter was subject to control of movement and deprivation of liberty, especially when such individual was also deemed by the provision of the Act to possess the right to self-discharge.

4.3.4. Implications-Control in Mental Health Services, Tension with Care?

The implications for these provisions lie in the role played by doctors, social workers, nurses and all other Approved Mental Health Practitioners who are mostly involved in applying the Act, by physically providing care for individuals in hospital and ensuring that treatment is managed within the legal provisions of the Act (Sullivan, 1998; CQC, 2013). Herein, lies the conflict, given that the role of these professionals is to provide care, they still must administer the legal framework of the Act which involves involuntary detention, deprivation of liberty, compulsion and coercion (Sullivan, 1998; Brown, 2016). The role of health professionals in acting as both protective gatekeepers towards preventing injuries to the clients who are experiencing mental illness while protecting members of the public from potential harm as a result of aggression or deviant behaviours at times necessitates the use of physical interventions (Prinsen & Delden, 2009) and other forms of control including seclusion, restraint and medications including rapid tranquilisation (CQC, 2013).

The fact that the coercive practice is considered necessary in order to correct real or potential harm to the client and/or others due to the adduced temporary mental incapacity of the client raises the legal, ethical and clinical complexity of situations (Sullivan, 1998; Prinsen & Delden, 2009). This results in a milieu of custody, supervision and control which make health professionals to be perceived as agents of control and coercion. This has been observed as creating a negative impact on the aims of providing care and creating and maintaining therapeutic relationship between the health professionals and the clients (Sullivan, 1998). In addition, in their bid to prevent harm and aggressive behaviour, health professionals apply the method of regular observation in the clinical area along with the other practices of seclusion and restraint in order to maintain an orderly condition in the environment for the safety of staff, clients, family, friends and visitors alike. This atmosphere of control has been described as surveillance, and deprivation of the liberty of the clients, which highlights further the conflict between helping the mentally ill and controlling them (Dennis, 1997; Duffy, 1995; Sullivan, 1998; Barber et al, 2012).

However, it has also been highlighted that although mental health clients may resent control, they also appreciate the need for some form of control in their lives, especially in their journey with mental illness (Schneider, 2010). It has been indicated that although they are deeply ambivalent about the control aspects of care, and whilst they find control highly dehumanising, as with their experience with coercion (Newton-Howes & Mullen, 2011) most of the time, they acknowledge that they sometimes also want and appreciate the control that is exercised over them to prevent behaviours that have in the past led to instability (Schneider, 2010; Newton-Howes & Mullen, 2011).

This indicates that there is a need for the professional to include the clients in all aspects of their care and make them active partners in decision making. However recent reports (CQC 2013:3) indicate that many clients are not involved in their care plans, nor are they aware of how to access support towards their recovery when they are discharged from acute hospital admissions. CQC (2013: 3) reports that:

> *"...more than a quarter (27%) of care plans showed no evidence of patients being involved in creating them. More than a fifth (22%) showed no evidence of patients' views being taken into account. This is no improvement on the previous year."*

4.3.5. Coercion in Mental Health Services - A Tool of Care?

> *"Interventions in care can be shown to be in the interest of patients, that is they can be seen as interventions for the attainment of autonomy instead of threatening autonomy"* (Verkerk, in Prinsen & Delden, 2009: 71).

Akin to the tension between care and control is the role played by the concept of coercion, which is demonstrated in the application of the provisions of the United Kingdom MHA, 1983 (as amended in 2007) (DoH, 2015), in the admission, treatment and management of the individuals who are considered to be suffering from mental illness in the community.

The idea behind coercion which is characterised by being forced or put under pressure to accept treatment for mental illness without the individual's consent, agreement or intention by applying powers as embedded in the provisions of the MHA (Newton-Howes, & Mullen, 2011). Coercion has been highlighted as a source of tension between the client's engagement with services and negative outcomes in relationship between professionals and clients (Newton-Howes & Mullen, 2011; Brown, 2016). This also further underlines the assertion that mental health theory and practice evolved due to tensions between diverse viewpoints concerning what causes mental illness problems and how best to respond to them and the people affected by them (Hardy, 2015). The MHA specified conditions under which individuals deemed to require involuntary psychiatric treatment can be detained. This includes such a person being suffering from a mental disorder, and that they need to receive suitable medical care for their own safety and the safety of other members of the public (Commission for Healthcare Audit and Inspection, 2007; Barber et al, 2012).

Human rights issues have arisen from decisions to detain under these provisions of the MHA, even as such detentions are usually combined with other coercive practices including restraint and seclusion (van Der Merwe, et al, 2009). The issue around mental capacity and the provisions of the Mental Capacity Act, MCA, (2005), also plays a role in this area, as principles are expected to be applied to protect the best interests of individuals who may be deemed to lack capacity in decision making (Brown, 2016). On discharge from acute care, mental health clients may also be subject to Community Treatment Orders (CTOs) under the MHA, which requires them to continue to receive treatment without their consent (Manning et al, 2011; Light et al, 2013).

Contemporary society holds strong views that mental health care involves detention and containment and other restraints on the actions and decisions of clients (O'Brien & Golding, 2003). These provision of the MHA impacts on the ability of the clients to play an equal role in decision making regarding their mental health, which has led to the assertion that "Judicial interventions such as community treatment orders can shift this balance of power, extending the possibility of compulsory treatment beyond the boundaries of hospitals, despite mixed evidence of effectiveness" (Newton-Howes & Mullen, 2011:465). O'Brien and Golding (2003: 67) also referred to these practices as "paternalistic" in nature as they are meant to be for the client's "own good".

The report by the Surgeon General on mental health in 1999 emphasized that:

> *"All services for those with a mental disorder should be consumer oriented and focused on promoting recovery. That is, the goal of services must not be limited to symptom reduction but should strive for restoration of a meaningful and productive life. Some people do not seek treatment because they are fearful of being forced to accept treatments not of their choice or of being treated involuntarily for prolonged periods"* (Newton-Howes, & Mullen, 2011: 465).

However, the provision of the MHA that includes 'sectioning', community treatment orders, seclusion and restraints all limits the autonomy of the mentally ill. It would appear that "there is a presupposition that because clients have limited autonomy, coercive practices are usually justified"; and that "There is considered to be prima facie right for mental health professionals to use coercive practices" (O'Brien & Golding 2003: 169). It has also been posited by Olsen (1998) in a quote by O'Brien and Golding (2003) that the motive behind the application of coercive practices is also not for the sole benefit of the clients but for the perceived benefit of others:

> *"Only psychiatric clients are routinely subjected to clinical interventions that they have specifically refused. Treatment is often forced on these clients for the benefit of others as well as themselves, further complicating ethical consideration* (Olsen 1998: 235)." (O'Brien and Golding, 2003: 169).

O'Brien and Golding (2003: 171) also highlight this, in agreement with a quote from Glenister (1997), regarding negative impact of coercion:

> *"....one of the therapeutic goals of mental healthcare is to develop autonomy in clients. Obviously, coercion can go directly against this .... Coercion also undermines the trust between clinician and client, which is harmful to the therapeutic relationship.* (Glenister 1997)". (O'Brien and Golding (2003: 171).

Diverse opinions have been raised regarding the concept of the autonomy of patients in healthcare settings and the ethical issues surrounding it, given that this trend towards more independence for patients has progressed in the last forty years and more, and led to what has been termed "a critique on a paternalistic approach to healthcare relationship" (Prinsen & Delden, 2009, p70). It has also been recalled that the advancement in the discourse towards patient autonomy had progressed from an increase in enlightenment and change in attitude to what constitutes "madness" (Prinsen & Delden, 2009).

The implications of this lie in the need for health professionals to balance their desire for the safety of their patients, staff and members of the public with the need to apply coercive practices (Prinsen & Delden, 2009; Sullivan, 1998). The consequence of what could be termed the patient-autonomy driven discourse has also been highlighted by Soloff, (1984), that: "social pressure toward greater freedom and less restrictive care push the psychiatrist to the limits of safety in managing the truly disturbed patients" (Prinsen &Delden, 2009: 70). This is like the challenges in social work where it has been highlighted that debates arise as to whether restrictive care "should be seen as a form of 'care', primarily concerned with individual wellbeing, or a form of 'control' contributing to the maintenance of social order" (Hardy, 2016: 12-13).

However, it has also been raised that the issue of autonomy should not be prioritised above other moral considerations including for example, beneficence (that is to act for the benefit of others). In this case, Prinsen & Delden (2009) highlighted the point raised by Beauchamp and Childress (2001) to the effect that autonomy should not be esteemed at the expense of respecting the social nature of persons and how their choices and actions can affect other people. In other words, respect for autonomy must not be seen to be "unduly legalistic (i.e. not highlighting legal rights and downplaying social practices" (Beauchamp & Childress, 2001: 70).

One other ethical issue regarding autonomy as it relates to health care and coercion lies in its relationship with moral values, which has been argued to be more important than autonomy (Prinsen & Delden, 2009). In following the assertion of Pellegrino and Campbell (Prinsen & Delden, 2009) in highlighting the relationship between autonomy on the one hand and dependency as a moral issue on the other, Prinsen & Delden (2009) asserted that dependency is more "fundamental than autonomy"(Prinsen and Delden, 2009:71). They expanded further on Campbell's argument that "a very independent individual could be lacking in autonomy in the sense that he cannot consistently exercise any degree of self-direction and cannot function as a member of society. Conversely, a dependent individual (e.g. a partner in a marriage) can still exercise autonomy" (Prinsen and Delden, 2009: 71). They stated further that the implication lies in the fact that coercive practices could not be dismissed on the platform of autonomy without considering the role played by ethical issues of relationships, morality and dependency.

This is further supported by Verkerk (2001) in exploring care ethics from the nature of care as a function of interdependency amongst humans; and the standpoint that autonomy should be considered in the context of responsibilities being higher than rights. Verkerk (2001:291) states that the "critique of autonomy in terms of self-sufficiency still leaves room for an idea of autonomy as the moral capacity to make one's own choices in life, sustained by others". Verkerk (2001: 291), therefore, advocates that "relational autonomy" and "compassionate interference" should be observed in psychiatric care.

A study involving clients living with schizophrenia has found that the tension between care and control presents complex dilemmas that must be negotiated by clients with schizophrenia in their daily lives (Schneider, 2010: 4). A study on the challenges faced by people living with mental illness in their interactions with housing authorities highlighted issues around control and coercion which played out in the requirements of the organisations to whom they have applied for housing (Schneider, 2010). It reported that some clients living with schizophrenia suggested that they risked housing services being withheld if they are not willing "to submit themselves to a variety of forms of which they regard as intrusive surveillance and coercive control over many (perhaps all) aspects of their lives" (Schneider, 2010: 4). They find that they are likely to put themselves in a state of jeopardy if they did not submit themselves to the so-called intrusive control and coercive practices by the service providers, as, if they are not willing to do this, they run the risk that care will be withheld (Schneider, 2010).

This risk of having care withheld by not adhering to coercive practices also highlights the imbalance of power within health and social care; as is indicated between the clients and the mental health practitioner, the negative impact on the former's right and autonomy to make decisions, which, in turn, negates the ethical principles required for protecting the rights of the individuals (O'Brien & Golding,

2003). It has been observed that the fact "that coercion can be flexibly interpreted, is applied both subjectively and objectively, poses a challenge to clarifying what constitutes subjectivity" (Newton-Howes, & Mullen, 2011: 465).

A systematic review of literature into coercion in psychiatry over a thirty-year period to 2009 conducted by Newton-Howes, and Mullen, (2011) underlined the experience and perception of mental health clients on action that leads to coercion as well as the challenges in reducing the impact of coercion in the lives of the clients. The review confirmed that "coercion is associated with negative concepts, such as feeling dehumanized and unheard" (Newton-Howes, & Mullen, 2011:469). The report also denied any idea of any positive theme resulting from the experience of coercion from the point of view of the clients, submitting that such positive topics suggesting any benefit from a coercive experience:

> *" ....tend to be based on patients' reflections some time after their inpatient experience, indicating a degree of understanding as to why an intervention was undertaken, rather than supporting the notion that patients do not see coercion in a negative way"* (Newton-Howes, & Mullen, 2011: 469).

This supports the assertion that although coercion is still being practiced as a necessity, and even deemed as unavoidable in many psychiatric settings (Torrey & Zdanowicz, 2001; McConnell & Gillett, 2006; O'Brien & Golding 2003; Muir-Cochrane, 2000), efforts need to be made to manage the experience of the clients in their encounter with health professionals in a way that promotes their autonomy whilst concurrently achieving positive outcome in their clinical experience and recovery (Newton-Howes, & Mullen, 2011; Barber et al, 2012; Brown, 2016).

This is, however, contrasted in reality with the recent findings by the CQC (2013) that coercive practices including seclusion, restraints and other restrictive actions continue to be applied in psychiatric settings in England, thereby leading to a negative impact on the therapeutic relationship between the health care staff and the clients. It was observed (Mind, 2013) that clinical ward rules that restrict the rights of patients include the practice of restraining or putting the patients into seclusion. Many are subjected to the use of prone or face down restraints. For example, statistics from a CQC (2013) report indicate that:

> *"prone or face-down restraint – defined as 'pinning and holding someone face down on the floor for a period of time' – had been used more than 3,000 times in NHS trusts in 2011/12" (CQC, 2013). This practice has been described as posing significant physical risks and dehumanising effects to the patients"* (CQC, 2013: 48).

Also, in their bid to deescalate situations where patients are judged to be posing danger to themselves, staff, and other members of the public, and to achieve environmental milieu, police are invited into psychiatric units to retrain patients (CQC, 2013). This has on occasions resulted in the use of Tasers, CS spray, and binding/tape and handcuffs (CQC, 2013). It has been observed that involving the police may be justified where healthcare staffs were incapable of managing challenging behaviours. However, it was asserted that: *"Police presence on wards can damage the therapeutic alliance between patients and staff"* (CQC, 2013: 51). The CQC also highlights the danger this practice potentially poses to maintaining control and restoring normalcy to the ward environment and the need to ensure that clear guidelines are in place to ensure where the police action starts and ends as well as clear processes that include the roles and expectations of all the relevant organisations involved (CQC, 2013).

4.4. The Relationship between Power, Control, Culture and Ethnicity

The concept of power has been found to be fundamental to culture, as well as perform functions that meet culturally applicable objectives (Torelli & Shavitt, 2010), as it has been found that "cultures nurture different views of what is desirable and meaningful to do with power" (Torelli & Shavitt, 2010: 73). This indicates that the identified collectivist and individualist cultures view power as a tool that is suitable for the advancement of the good of all in the society and personal benefits respectively. It also indicates that power and control are dictated by dominant culture in the same vein that dominant power could dictate cultures (Torelli & Shavitt, 2010).

Considering the relationship of power and control on culture, and vice versa, with focus on the collectivist society, it would suggest that there are various implications:

- Dominant cultures-induced power- that is power that is derivable from discourses of the dominant majority has the tendency to encourage and perpetuate marginalisation of the minority in the society. In contrast, however, cultures that regard power to be used for the collective benefit of the society will tend to promote a more egalitarian society which would care for all members of the society (Torelli & Shavitt, 2010).
- Perceived helplessness becomes ingrained in the minority population due to the influence of the majority induced discourses (Torelli & Shavitt, 2010);
- The feeling of subjugation may result in learned helplessness, which becomes the coping strategy for the conditions;
- This may in turn lead to inaction or passivity by the minority;
- Individuals from the collectivist culture may also be prone to accepting the control exerted by the majority discourses which emanated from individualist culture induced power, which consequently becomes a learned behaviour;
- This suggests that the form of control exerted by dominant cultures becomes acceptable by the minority groups. This suggests that it may lead to inaction from the minority cultures as a form of acceptance.

It would suggest that members of a collectivist culture that is in the minority in a society dominated by individualist culture could, therefore, be subject to double jeopardy – on the one hand, the collectivist culture that is in the minority has no power and can, therefore, not follow through on the nature, intent and purpose of the culture, that is to look for the good of all its membership (Foucault, 1980, 2010).

On the other hand, since the collectivist culture is found to be dominated by the populous individualist culture that has the power (because they are in the majority and therefore exerts control), the member of the collectivist culture would have no choice than to as it were, 'toe the line' as may be required by the individualistic culture-induced rules and norms which by nature focuses more on the rights, prestige and achievements of the individual. This may also lead to the acceptance of the status quo due to a feeling of hopeless and helpless perception that the collectivist member may have that it has no ability to demand or enforce any changes. Also, given that members of the collectivist society tend to subscribe to acceptance of some level of LOC – that is, agreeing to relinquishing rights or control (Cheng et al, 2013), this may be highly exacerbated by the dominance of the power derived and controlled by individualist orientation.

4.4.1. Summary & Implications of Power, Control for BME Mental Health

This leads to the implication of the perception of control from the point of view of the mental health clients from ethnic minority cultures.

As the clients are controlled by the power exerted by the MHA in the provisions of Involuntary Treatment Order (ITO) and Community Treatment Order (CTO), the clients may perceive a feeling of becoming rendered powerless from these provisions, as their opinion has minimal impact on a statutory regulation which has already been promulgated and passed without the input or opinion of the clients. The clients find that they must comply with regulation, including the attendant use of coercion that emanated from the power and control of the MHA, which originated from individualist orientated and majority dominant discourse (Torelli & Shavitt, 2010). This disempowerment may also impact on the level of trust in the system.

The role of the professional can also be viewed by the clients as that of an agent of the statutory compliance rather than as a professional who wants to help the clients to achieve recovery from mental illness (Schneider, 2010), which could make it counterproductive. Another issue lies in the fact that the Act adopts a 'one size fits all' approach to mental illness in the society and has not considered social and cultural indicators or personal circumstances of the mentally ill clientele (Fernando & Keating, 2009; Fernando, 1998) especially those from the collectivist cultures.

Although it may not be entirely valid that all BME groups subscribe to the concept of collectivist cultures, studies have indicated that Individuals from BME community are predominantly from a collectivist culture (Cheng et al, 2013). It means, therefore, that clients from the BME background are likely to "accept" dominant power as a given/norm and may not protest its dominance. This comes from a feeling or perception of powerlessness due to minority status, as well as the cultural tendency to accept the norm, and not make any effort to change the conditions. This could be linked to disillusionment, a feeling of disempowerment with mental health services without any corresponding resistant action other than to withdraw from, avoid engagement with, as well as become totally passive and apathetic to the services.

In addition, the Act that is perceived by the BME community member to have been a product of an individualist orientation may lead to the reaction of hopeless and helplessness, since:

- It suggests that the MHA legislation comes from the dominant culture that is different in nature to the collectivist culture were not originally designed to meet the needs of the collectivist community member who would expect that health is the collective responsibility of all members of the community (Cheng et al, 2013). Consequently, the BME clients would expect that his/her health challenges can be managed with the active involvement and support of the members of his/her family and community. However, as the legislation and practices that came as an offshoot of the MHA (2007) promotes individualist culture, this means that it would be highly unsuitable for the BME clients, especially given that in practice the whole pre, during and post intervention processes including admission, intervention, assessment processes, diagnosis, treatment and discharge management are based on individualist orientation and hardly involves members of the immediate family of the Service users, let alone the community at large.

- It suggests a tendency for the BME community member who comes from the collectivist persuasion to agree to accept some level of control in contrast to the member of the individualist orientation (Cheng et al, 2013). This would suggest that the BME client is not likely to protest any perceived inadequacies in the system or unsuitable treatment or experience from the individualist powered MH Act, but rather accept the situation as the condition that he/she can manage within the constraints provided by the system. This is one of the negative indicators that arise from the perceived "benefit" of LOC to the collectivist society.
- It highlights the importance of intercultural sensitivity, like what has been posited by Bennet (1993); sensitivity between cultures should be developed. This suggests that there is a need for health and social care services that seek to engage the BME community member to demonstrate the following understanding:
    - Given that the current legislation and services are based on individualist orientation, the services and practitioners need to recognise that the BME comes from different cultural backgrounds and the likelihood that specific expectations may be held by them from their respective view and interpretation of internal and external control
    - Based on the origin of this legislation and services, that the BME community members' interpretation of

power, control, and the expectations resulting from these would impact on their perception of mental wellbeing and their response to, engagement with and overall decision to embrace the mental health service as an institution that is interested in their recovery from mental illness and achieving their optimum wellbeing. This raises the importance of the issue of LOC from the point of view of the BME clients and the need to explore it further as it relates to their experience with the mental health services and social care.

4.4.2. Conclusion-Implications for African and Caribbean Mental Health

The various safeguards indicated in various legislations and institutions including the MHA (1983, 2007); the Mental Capacity Act (2005); the Deprivation of Liberty Safeguards, the Human Rights Act (1998) and the European Convention on Human Rights, are set up to protect the rights of the clients in their mental health challenges. It also indicates that these provisions are aimed at ensuring that the concepts discussed in this chapter including care, coercion, control and power are not applied to abuse the rights of clients but are applied by public authorities, including health professionals, institutions such as the CQC, policy makers, and all stakeholders in the best interest of the clients and the public.

However, the observed problems and challenges including the over representation of members of the BME communities in mental health settings, coercive practices, dissatisfaction with services and other challenges as indicated in chapter one of this thesis, continue to exist. It would, therefore, suggest that these provisions have not impacted positively on the experiences of BME service users, especially the A & C groups, thereby calling into question whether the provisions were made by considering the collectivist orientations of these groups and their implications for their mental health challenges. It would also suggest that the failure or lack of impact on the status quo of the BME mental health profile could be due to the individualist orientation of these provisions, which means that the provisions and needs of groups of collectivist culture have been ignored. It further indicates the desirability of exploring how these individualist originated provisions could be amended to cater for the needs of the collectivist groups in the society, which the A & C communities belong, in order to achieve better mental health outcomes for them.

4.5. Summary Qualification- Other Areas of Elements of Mental Health and Social Care Not Covered in This Study

This section of the review of literature has explored power, care, control and coercion in mental health services. The review has, however, not covered forensic and judicial system related mental health care, and its implications for the tension between care and control, as they are not the focus of this study.

In addition, it has been deliberately decided to omit the concepts of care, control and coercion in relation to social care, especially in areas relating to children, families and vulnerable adults. Other areas omitted include children in care in mental health settings, the experiences of families involved in children taken into care as well as the mental health implications. The experiences of BME people in children welfare issues, children taken into care, the experiences of parents, and in particular the experiences of A & C groups in relation to children in care experiences, including the children as well as the parents are also not included. This is due to the understanding that these areas are wide in coverage and this study will not be able to accord the issues enough attention for in-depth exploration, and the author has decided to explore these issues in future studies.

5| The Study

5.1. Focus of Study

The literature review in chapter 4 has resulted in the identification of various gaps in knowledge in the relationship between culture and ethnicity and the concept of Locus of Control in relation to the tension between care and control, and the role of the accompanying concepts including coercion and power in mental health, as it relates to the Black and Minority Ethnic (BME) peoples.

In view of the multifaceted nature of the research gaps identified in the literature review, it was decided with guidance from supervision that this study should focus on exploring the first four items described in the gaps in knowledge section. It was also decided to explore these areas from the perspective of the BME sub cultural groups of the African and Caribbean populations. The areas of investigation include:

- The perspectives of Locus of Control (LOC) of the African and Caribbean (A & C) mental health service users in general and mental health contexts;
- Relationship between culture, ethnicity and the locus of control orientation of A & C mental health service users, in the context of their experiences with mental health services.

The main objective of this study was to advance understanding of the relationship between locus of control and the tension between care and control in the experiences of A & C service users. The decision to commence investigation into the LOC of the A and C mental health service users in both mental health and general contexts was with a view to addressing the research gap that relates to the need to investigate the perspectives of LOC of the A & C groups. Literature also suggests that an understanding of their perspectives could provide insights into how mental health clients can be influenced by various agents of internal and external control (Cheng et al, 2013; Declerck et al, 2006). It has also been suggested that the perspectives of clients must be paramount in investigating their experiences with health services (Bhui et al, 2013). It was also aimed at addressing the gap in knowledge by investigating their LOC orientation from the context of their experiences of mental illness, as it has been observed that carrying out investigations from the perspectives of clients are beneficial towards improving their engagement with services (Treacy et al, 2015). It was also decided that carrying out these investigations can provide foundation knowledge for the observed challenges of BME mental health by investigating LOC from the experiences of A & C groups and provide opportunity to explore other observed gaps in the future.

The choice of the A & C populations was also due to the over-representation of these groups (as sub groups of BME populations) in Mental Health Services (MHS) as has been indicated in chapter one, the literature review and subsequent chapters in this study. The indicated areas of focus were also aimed to be investigated using some specific research questions to be explored with the participants, which informed the study design and methods (Yardley & Bishop, 2015).

The focus on these areas is also intended to achieve the aims and objectives of this study- to explore the experiences of the A & C groups in relation to these concepts of LOC, care, control, culture, ethnicity and other concepts, in order to increase our understanding towards addressing the challenges and improving the mental health profile of the A & C groups in England.

5.2. Research Questions

The research questions designed from the literature review and theoretical framework could be explored from the experiences and views of key stakeholders as participants (Cheng et al, 2013). This includes mental health clients, family, carers and health professionals (as deemed applicable).

However, it has been decided for the purpose of this study to explore the questions from the perspectives of the A & C clients only. The reasons for this approach are three-fold, the first being the over-representation of the population in mental health services. The second is due to the observation that investigations of this nature have been seldom, if not rarely, explored from the clients' perspectives. It is also with a view to giving the clients a voice, as they are the most disaffected stakeholders who are at the receiving end of mental health services in the United Kingdom (McKenzie & Bhui, 2007; Bhui et al, 2013).

The following research questions have informed the methods that have been used in conducting this study:

- What are the perspectives and understanding of Locus of Control (LOC) of A & C mental health service users in general?
- What are the perspectives and understanding of LOC of A & C mental health service users in mental health context?
- Is there any relationship between culture and the LOC of the A & C service users in their experiences with mental health services?
- How could this understanding around culture and LOC be used to improve mental health services for African and African-Caribbean service users?

5.3. Choice of Paradigm in Healthcare Research

> *"In the context of health care research, a researcher's paradigmatic positioning relates to their understanding of the nature of knowledge (their epistemological standpoint) and of reality (their ontological standpoint)".* (Broom and Willis, 2007:17)

It has been observed that research in health care has historically taken varying epistemological and ontological standpoints, which, in turn, not only dictates the objective and design of the studies, but also impacts on the knowledge produced there from (Broom and Willis,

2007). Healthcare researchers have also traditionally embraced paradigms, although it has been reported that "The commonest split has been between the positivists and the constructivists in their choices of paradigm" (Broom & Willis, 2007: 18).

It has also been stated that the greatest research outcomes can be achieved by taking a variety of paradigmatic positions (Broom & Willis, 2007). The aim must be to endeavour to identify the best method that offers an opportunity to explore and research queries, which may include the use of a combination of methods and/or paradigms (Broom & Willis, 2007). However, the philosophical standpoint needs to be reflected in the results and analysis, as "ontologically speaking, social reality cannot be both objectivist (positivist) in nature and also a social construction (constructionist/interpretivist)" (Broom & Willis, 2007: 18).

Any perceived flaws in the results of health care studies are thus impacted by the choice of paradigm, even as it has been asserted that "Much research into health has often failed to understand inequalities within a complex social world" (Bergin et al, 2008: 172). In their discuss of the importance of paradigm in nursing research, Weaver and Olson (2005), advocate a variety of methods that conserve the individual theoretical viewpoints of each model and that "situating research within paradigms, as well as the knowledge resulting from research processes, must be considered in the light of their ability to advance the social mission of nursing: to enhance health and wellbeing and alleviate suffering" (Weaver & Olson, 2005: 466).

In highlighting perceived weaknesses in the philosophy behind positivism and constructivism and the research relating to inequalities in mental health, Bergin et al (2008), also stated that "Because of the philosophical constraints of positivism and constructivism, factors that are often invisible to existence, not capable of being measured or not expressed by the researched are quite often missed during the research process" (Bergin et al, 2008: 173). In addition, a critique of positivism lies in the fact that it "is defined by its ontological construction of the world – empirical observation; and by its epistemological perspective on that world – that things only exist if they are observable or measurable" (Wainwright & Forbes, 2000: 264). On the other hand, the criticism of interpretivism lies in "their ontological construction of the social world that is limited to the conscious interpretations of the social actors of interest" (Wainwright & Forbes, 2000: 268).

It has been suggested that researchers need to focus more on the fact that different epistemological standpoints offer different views on how people see and relate with the world, rather than being distracted by arguments related to their different opinions (Evans et al, 2010). Cohen and Dennett (2011) highlight the subjectivity of the human experience, due to the influence of social, cultural, political and environmental factors, which, in turn, impact on their view of the world. As individual's consciousness cannot be separated from their function, it is, therefore, important to draw interpretations from the meaning individuals perceive from their subjective human experiences (Cohen & Dennett, 2011). The qualitative methodology adopted for this study are in line with the interpretive/constructionist paradigm due to its applicability and suitability to health care research, which is a focus of this study on the one hand, and a desire to conduct make meaning of healthcare experiences of service users.

5.4. Inclination to Interpretivism for This Study

> *"...the premise of interpretive researchers is that access to reality (whether given or socially constructed) is only through social constructions such as language, consciousness and shared meanings ... Interpretive paradigm is underpinned by observation and interpretation, thus to observe is to collect information about events, while to interpret is to make meaning of that information by drawing inferences or by judging the match between the information and some abstract pattern.... It attempts to understand phenomena through the meanings that people assign to them"* (Thomas, 2010: 296).

This section explains the inclination towards interpretivism for this qualitative study, including why and how it was applied, including a discussion of the identified critique and limitations indicated in the earlier section. Denzin and Lincoln (2005) asserted that 'qualitative research is endlessly creative and interpretive', and that 'qualitative interpretations are constructed' (Denzin and Lincoln, 2005: 26). In addition, as indicated in the above quote from Thomas (2010), issues can be understood by drawing from the meaning that individuals make of them (Thomas, 2010). The interpretive component of the qualitative research has also been described as a process that involves the movement of information received by the researcher to a 'recreated' text, as a 'working interpretive document that contains the writer's attempt to make sense of what he or she has learned.' (Denzin and Lincoln, 2005: 26). In the light of the importance of drawing interpretation of people's perceptions highlighted in the previous section on paradigm in healthcare research, interpretivism was considered the most suitable paradigm for this study, as it offered the prospect of enabling the researcher apply the perceptions of the participants from their experiences to arrive at the meaning they make of such experiences and their world view (Denzin & Lincoln, 2005; Cohen & Dennett, 2011). It includes the process of description of such views and experiences and drawing an interpretation from such views.

Creswell (2009) posits that ideas and perceptions can be understood from the meaning that develops from the description and interpretation of the textual material obtained by researcher from the study participants. This was applicable to this study, as the researcher relied on the participants' perceptions to draw meanings from their decision making to create new understanding regarding their LOC orientation in both general and mental health contexts. In addition, as indicated earlier, the interpretivist paradigm favours the use of qualitative research (Weaver & Olson, 2005; Broom & Wills, 2007), which is applicable for this study, which is based on one-to-one interviews and focus groups.

Thomas (2010), asserted that inquiries can be conducted through interpretivism in order to understand "the nature or qualities of complex social group behaviours by employing interpretive and naturalistic approaches.....and takes into account the unperturbed views of the participants as the purpose is generally to aim for objectivity....to become more familiar with the phenomenon of interest, to achieve a deep understanding of how people think about a topic and to describe in great detail the perspectives of the research participants" (Thomas, 2010: 306). Furthermore, as explained under Interpretive Phenomenological Analysis (IPA) in the analysis section (3.8 Analysis of data) in this report, interpretivism was also adopted in combination with the IPA approach adopted for the analysis of this study, as it also aligns favourably with understanding phenomenological approaches (Fade, 2004; Smith et al, 2012). This inclination was also due to the observation that IPA is rooted in the theoretical underpinnings of interpretivism, which is based on the premise that human conceptualisation and views of reality (world view) can be multifaceted and different, and are dictated by their understanding, view or interpretation of their experiences (Fade, 2004; Smith et al, 2012). IPA also aligns more appropriately with achieving the aims of Interpretivism in this study in contrast to grounded theory due to the latter's disposition towards positivist paradigm (Charmaz, 2000). Discourse analysis was also considered in view of its link with generation of knowledge (Foucault, 1972). However, IPA favours a more flexible approach to interpretation than discourse analysis, which is necessary for this study (Charmaz, 2000).

Interpretivism was also used as it offered an opportunity to explore views of service users based on their experiences, which cannot be objectively measured. This presented a more suitable alternative to a positivist ontological approach which relies on empirical observation and measurement, which results in issues that are not capable of being observed or measured being missed (Wainwright & Forbes, 2000; Bergin et al, 2008). By asking study participants questions in relation to their LOC in general and mental health contexts, the researcher was able to use interpretivism to explore their understanding and perception of the concept from their experiences, which cannot be measured or quantified into figures.

The participants' experiences could also not be measured, as they were based on their past experiences, which could not have been possible with a positivist approach. In addition, interpretivism has been suggested as a more suitable approach in exploring issues relating to health inequalities, particularly inequalities in mental health (Bergin et al, 2008), which is applicable to this study. By asking the study participants questions relating to their LOC, particularly on issues relating to their perception of control over their lives, the researcher was able to obtain information relating to how they perceived their LOC were impacted by their experiences in general and mental health contexts, issues that impact on their experiences, and their interpretation of such experiences. These viewpoints from the social world of the study participants could not have been easily obtained by objective measurement via a positivist approach.

Although interpretivism has been criticised for having a weakness of basing its ontological construction on the conscious interpretation that study participants make of their social world (Wainwright & Forbes, 2000) as opposed to measurement and observations, interpretivism was still considered more suitable for this study into human experiences that cannot be objectively quantified, but has to be based on what has been described as a 'reconstructed understandings of the social world' (Denzin & Lincoln, 2005: 184).

This is since human experiences are liable to be subjective as they are impacted by social, environmental, cultural and political factors (Cohen and Dennett, 2011). These factors are applicable to this study, as the inequalities in mental health that applies to the study participants, are also impacted by these factors, and could be explored using interpretivism, by asking the study participants to make sense of their world as they are affected by the factors in their experiences. For example, as one of the objectives of the study was to explore LOC within the context of culture from the study participants, interpretivism was more applicable for this study, as it was used to gain understanding of the participants' view of the relationship between culture and their LOC, which could not have been objectively deciphered by observation and measurement using a positivist approach.

5.5. Methods Adopted for the Collection of Data- Qualitative Approach

> *"....qualitative research is a means for exploring and understanding the meaning individuals or groups ascribe to a social or human problem"* (Creswell, 2009: 4*).*

Considering the interpretive approach adopted for this study, a qualitative approach was also adopted in the collection of data, in a bid to obtain answers to the research questions (Thanh & Thanh, 2015; Thomas, 2010). A link has been made between a qualitative research approach and interpretivist paradigm (Thanh & Thanh, 2015; Thomas, 2010; Denzin & Lincoln, 2005). Thanh and Thanh (2015) suggest that: "There is a tight connection between interpretivist paradigm and qualitative methodology as one is a methodological approach and one is a means in collecting data.

Researchers who are using interpretivist paradigm and qualitative methods often seek experiences, understandings and perceptions of individuals for their data to uncover reality rather than rely on numbers of statistics" (Thanh & Thanh, 2015: 24). This is applicable to this study, as the research questions seek to understand LOC from the perspectives of service users, based on their experiences, using semi structured interview questions in individual and focus group settings (Maxwell, 2005; Seale, 2006). This is in contrast with quantitative methods which involve the collection of data via the use of questionnaires, surveys, the conduct of experiments, and use of documentary as well as observation methods (Maxwell, 2005; Seale, 2006).

The inclination towards a qualitative approach in data collection was also formed from the interest in this study to evaluate the perceptions of study participants based on their experiences rather than relying on numbers or statistics that emanate from quantitative approaches (Thanh & Thanh, 2015; Yardley & Bishop, 2015). A qualitative approach has also been credited with the ability to enable researchers to find solutions to health care policy problems which can be suggested to impact government policies.

Qualitative research can also enable researchers to 'isolate target populations, show immediate effects of certain programs on such groups, and isolate the constraints that operate against policy changes in such settings' (Denzin & Lincoln, 2005: 26). This is also applicable to this study, as it is envisaged that the findings from the service users' perspectives on their LOC and their mental health experiences might contain suggestions that could impact government policies in relation to A & C mental health. This is in view of the findings from the literature review regarding past government policies aimed at addressing mental health inequalities in relation to BME mental health such as the Delivering Race Equality (DRE) (DoH, 2005). The DRE was found to have had minimal impact on the mental health inequalities (Crisp et al, 2016), as highly disproportionate rate of admissions and compulsory detention experienced by the BME groups, including A & C peoples in England continued to be observed (Care Quality Commission, 2011; Crisp et al, 2016).

5.5.1. Strategy Applied for Exploring the Research Questions

This section discusses the strategy applied in exploring the research questions for this study. It includes a description of the specific qualitative tools applied, including the interview schedule and focus group guide. The responses to the semi structured questions and conversations held with the study participants on LOC during the one-to-one interviews and focus group sessions formed the basis of the qualitative data collected to answer the first question for this study. The first research question was aimed at assessing the participants' idea regarding control over their lives, and the extent to which they felt that they were in control in general. The second question relating to the mental health LOC of the participants was also explored within the semi structured interview schedule and focus group guide to assess both the participants' perspectives on general LOC and mental health LOC during the one-to-one and focus group sessions.

The third question was designed to examine the study participants' views regarding their LOC and their ethnicity and culture in mental health context.

The fourth research question was designed to enable the study participants to express how their own perspective and understanding of their LOC and the two other questions relating to both general and mental health contexts as well as their ethnicity and cultural perspectives could be applied to improve mental health experiences for the A & C populations. The questions were explored within the qualitative method by adopting the application of a high level of flexibility to encourage conversations with the study participants to reflect on their responses to the questions that have been explored in the first three research questions.

It was also aimed at enabling them to express their suggestions on the way forward to improve mental health services for the members of their community and the BME groups. It was also envisaged that the study participants would be able to share their reflections on the questions and indicate their views on how the interplay of ethnicity, culture, LOC orientation, and any other issues that might have arisen in the interview sessions could be addressed by all stakeholders to improve the current statistics and profile of the mental health of the subject population.

5.5.2. Qualitative Tools Applied- One-to-One Interviews and Focus Groups

The conduct of one-to-one interview and focus groups sessions in which semi structured interview questions were administered, have been adopted in order to explore LOC from the experiences, perspectives and opinions of the study participants in relation to the research questions in both general and mental health contexts. This two-pronged approach of combining focus groups and one-to one interview was also adopted in order to take advantage of the benefits as well as minimise the impact of the demerits of both approaches (Lambert & Loiselle, 2007).

One-to-one interviews are suitable in eliciting detailed information that can enable gathering of context-based data relating to the subject matter of culture's influence on the participants' perception of control in relation to the research questions (Williams & Katz, 2001). Focus group sessions were also held in order to provide a safe space for each participant to share their views with people with similar experiences of treatment by mental health services, including hospitalisation in psychiatric settings and experience with community mental health teams (Williams & Katz, 2001). A focus group has been defined as "a small gathering of individuals who have a common interest or characteristic, assembled by a moderator, who uses the group and its interactions as a way to gain information about a particular issue" (Williams & Katz, 2001: 2).

Williams and Katz (2001) also support the inclination towards focus group interview as a different method of generating data by encouraging both individual and collective responses to the questions from different perspectives. Earlier submissions assert that focus groups method offers the benefit of encouraging individuals who may not like to be interviewed individually. It also limits the discrimination that could be experienced or perceived by participants who have difficulties in reading and writing, as they are given the opportunity to express their views verbally (Kitzinger, 1995). Focus group interviews may also encourage individuals who may feel that they have no idea or are unable to make contribution to discussions to engage more in discussions, thereby enabling more information to be obtained from them than through individual interviews (Kitzinger, 1995). In addition, focus groups are also a tool that can enable the collection of large data as well as enrichment of information (Stewart & Shamdasani, 1990).

Focus groups also provide an environment whereby the study participants 'influence and are influenced' (Krueger & Casey, 2000), and where the role of the researcher includes "that of moderator, listener, observer, and eventually inductive analyst" (Williams & Katz,

2001: 2). This was also applicable to this study, in addition to a deliberate attempt made by the researcher to exercise a degree of flexibility in order to allow for the inclusion of additional participants if necessary (Willig, 2003). The focus group sessions were also favoured in order to achieve the benefits of "increased number of participants, observable dynamic interactions, and cost-effectiveness" (Papadakis &Carolissen, 2012: 668).

In the light of the understanding of focus groups, concerted efforts were made by the interviewer to limit the potential drawbacks of the focus groups, which include interview bias and the likelihood of individual voices being silenced in a group situation (Kitzinger, 1995). The assertion by Stewart and Shamdasani (1990) suggest that generalisation could not be applied to specific population as each focus group is considered a unique set of opinion. This observation was anticipated to be countered in this study by adding the complimentary tool of individual interviews.

The focus groups sessions were moderated by the researcher introducing specific aspects of the questions with a view to ensuring that every focus group member was heard, and that group member's conversations were focused on the main purpose of the study.

The moderation also involved asking additional questions for further clarification, observing the atmosphere and interaction among participants and making brief notes regarding the two sessions. Furthermore, in line with recommendations about focus group management (Willig, 2003; Starks & Trinidad, 2007); the researcher did not rely on nods or monosyllabic responses but also asked follow-up questions to ensure the information was understood by all the participants. It has also been found that combining individual interview and focus group data leads to both complimentary and overlapping findings that can contribute to 'a coherent and more nuanced understanding' of phenomenon being studied (Lambert & Loiselle, 2007: 234).

5.5.3. Interview Schedules, Pilot and Conduct of Interviews

Two interview schedules were developed for this study, one for the one-to-one interview and the other a guide for the focus groups (Appendices 2 and 3). The questions used for this study were piloted with a group of four African and Caribbean mental health services clients, who provided feedback on the content and structure of the questions. It has been asserted that pilot study is used in social science research to determine the extent to which an instrument could be feasible, as well as to run a pre-test of a research tool (Teijlingen & Hundley, 2002). Other reasons have been adduced for conducting pilot of instruments, including ascertaining the adequacy of a tool, designing a suitable, realistic procedure for research and likelihood that a research approach could be successful (Arain et al, 2010; Thabane et al, 2010). The comments were solicited by the researcher in order to not only find out which of the questions the participants might not feel comfortable to respond to, but also to prevent researcher bias and promote reliability of the data (Thabane et al, 2010). The opinions expressed by the four A & C service users were incorporated into the final version of the two sets of questions designed and used for the study.

The questions in the two schedules were also designed by the researcher with advice and guidance from the supervisor, to meet the aims of the study and were in line with the research questions of exploring understanding of LOC within the study population. They were principally aimed at eliciting interviewees' perception of LOC by drawing on their personal understanding, opinions and experiences of mental health services, from the domain of culture, control, care, power and coercion. The questions also sought to discover from the clients' personal approaches to control, decision making in their lives, the extent to which they rely on others before they take important decisions. For example, one of the questions (in the one-to-one interview schedule), states: *"How do you make decisions about important things in your life?"*

Other questions were designed to discover how the interviewees respond to control over them, their understanding of power, coercion, care and control, the existence of any link between these concepts and culture as well as their experiences with mental health services, and how the services they used had been impacted by these concepts and/or vice versa.

Following a successful pilot, the interviews were conducted by the researcher. Particular attention was paid by the researcher to the interviewees' responses to the semi structured questions. He also asked additional follow-up questions at points where he felt that it was necessary to further explore the interviewee's responses to questions (Smith & Osborne, 2003; Borkoles et al, 2008; Gillard et al, 2015).

This approach was used throughout the interviews in order to make sure that the interviewees were comfortable to express their opinions, share their experiences as well as have some ownership of the interview session. The one-to-one interviews were conducted in quiet rooms which allowed for ease of audio tape recording following interviewees' consent, with appropriate heating and the interviewees were provided beverages and water to ensure that they were comfortable during the approximately 90 minutes period of interviews. The interviews were transcribed verbatim following the recordings.

5.6. Study Setting and Participants- BME & A &C Population and Service Users in South London

With a population of 1.45 million, the southern part London in which this study was conducted, is growing at one of the fastest rates of any region in England (National Health Service, NHS, South West London Collaborative Commissioning) (2014). The population is projected to increase to 1,647,200 by 2030 (South East Public Health Observatory, SEPHO, 2011).

The proportion of the population in the South London Boroughs (from which the sample of this study was taken), which is from Black and Minority Ethnic groups is estimated to be 18.8% (Office of National Statistics, ONS, 2009). Ethnicity estimated in 2009 for South London has 7.3% of its population in the most deprived national quintile and 20.8% of the population in the least deprived quintile, which indicates that there is a low socio-economic status. A more recent statistics from the 2011 Census indicates a major increase in the proportion of BME population living in the south London Boroughs (ONS, 2012).

However, the boroughs in which this study is undertaken had over 45% of its population in the most deprived quintile (Department of Communities and Local Government) (DCLG), 2010). The Black population (including 'Black and Black Caribbean', 'African' and 'Black other') is estimated at 8.1 percent of the Borough population in 2009 (ONS, 2011), while the latest 2011 census report indicated that "the proportion of Black/African/Caribbean/Black British residents (10.6%) was greater than the national average (3.4%), but less than the proportion across London (13.3%)". (ONS, 2012)

Mental health services in this South London Borough are provided by a local Mental Health Trust. It was reported in 2013 that "Black and African-Caribbean patients continue to be overrepresented among the detained patient population compared with local population profiles" (CQC, 2013). The 2013 report also indicated that in comparison to 10.6 per cent of the general population being made up of this ethnic group in this Borough, more than 31 per cent the patients detained under the MHA were 'Black or African-Caribbean'. This formed the basis of concentrating on the A & C mental health clients for this study.

The participants for this study have been chosen from this South London Borough due to the researcher's familiarity with this borough from a period working at a local University with some exposure to the Borough's mental health profile. This has led to the awareness of the fact that this Borough has a high proportion of BME residents and one of the highest A & C groups in mental health settings compared to the national average (ONS, 2012). The percentage break down of aggregated ethnic groups across the general population in the chosen south London Borough, shows 51% White British, 14% Asian and 10% Black African, British, and Caribbean (CQC, 2013). The percentage of the ethnic groups detained under Section 136 of the Mental Health Act in the Borough in 2013-2014 also indicates that peoples of Black British, African, Caribbean, Other made up 35% of the detentions. This suggests that although the Black, Caribbean, Other population accounted for 10 per cent of the Borough's population (ONS, 2012), this same group accounted for a high percentage of Section 136 detentions in years 2013-2014 (CQC, 2013). Section 136 of the Mental Health Act gives power to the Police to detain someone suspected of suffering from mental Illness to be detained for assessment and treatment.

5.6.1. Data Collection –Inclusion Criteria, Sampling and Access

This study was based within community setting. Local charitable organisations that provide support and socialisation projects to mental health service users from BME backgrounds in south London were approached in writing and by personal contact by the researcher for permission to access their organisations and approach the target population for participation in the study. This was intended to gain in-depth perspectives from the participants in both individual and group contexts, and to minimise the demerits of both individual and focus group methods explained under qualitative tools applied.

Following permission by the coordinators of the charity organisations and introduction to potential participants who consented to taking part, the conduct of one-to-one interviews and focus group sessions were carried out within the premises of the charity organisations as they were easily accessible and convenient for the participants. The participants were already familiar with the locations due to regularly attending the charities for recreational, educational and socialisation purposes. The locations also offered a conducive and comfortable environment to conduct focus group sessions with people they had been sharing activities with, in the community.

5.6.1.1. Inclusion Criteria

Participants were included in this study if they were:

- Male or female aged between 18 and 65 from the A & C populations – born in the United Kingdom, in the Caribbean, Africa, or elsewhere, who described him/herself as being of African and/or Caribbean origin;
- Mental health clients with a diagnosis of a mental disorder who had been discharged from psychiatric hospitals and was recovering in the community;
- Clients who were attending the drop-in services of local charity organisations, or who were living in supported or privately rented accommodation in the community.
- Clients who were able to understand the contents of the research information package and consent requirements;
- Clients who were to be considered sufficiently stable in terms of their mental health and capable of providing informed consent to participate in a 60 minute or longer period of one-one interviews or focus group interviews and were able to respond to the questions in English. This was determined with the support of the managers and members of staff of the community organisations who were familiar with and had been providing services to the participants.

5.6.1.2. Exclusion Criteria

Mental health clients were excluded from the enquiry if they were not of African or African Caribbean origin; in psychotic state; under 18 years of age and over 65; had a diagnosis of dementia, as this condition affects an individual's ability to give a full opinion. Clients with other organic brain disorders, learning disability and other co morbidity that could interfere with their participation in the one-to-one and focus group interviews were also excluded; as it was considered that these conditions were likely to impact on their participation and results.

5.6.2. Purposive Sampling

After determination of the inclusion and exclusion criteria for the study participants, a purposive sampling method was applied in the data collection for this study. Purposive sampling has been defined as a non-probability sampling method by which study participants are selected from a population based on specific features and the objective of the study. Purposive sampling is also known as judgmental sampling, as it relies on the judgement of the researcher and how they perceive that their research objectives can be achieved by focusing on deciding individuals to be included in research based on specific criteria (Palys, 2008; Palinkas et al, 2015). This technique is also based on criteria determined by the researcher and is favoured in qualitative research in order to achieve richness of information (Bernard, 2002; Palinkas et al, 2015). This type of sampling method is also suitable for identifying and selecting individuals who have experienced specific phenomenon being investigated (Palinkas et al, 2015; Cresswell& Plano, 2011). This condition is applicable to this study, as it involves identification and selection of individuals with experience of mental illness and mental health services, which is the focus of this study. This characteristic of homogenous sampling is also understood to favour eliciting and obtaining necessary perception by providing appropriate contexts of inquiry (Oliver, 2006; Palys, 2008; Smith & Osborn, 2003).

Following liaison with and consent of the organisers and coordinators of the charity organisations, and group leaders of various activities (including arts and crafts, drawings, dance sessions, Bingo sessions, table tennis and pool games), the researcher conversed with several groups of individuals at the start, during and after several drop-in activities. The researcher invited interested individuals to participate by explaining the purpose of the study, the inclusion criteria, voluntary participation, as well as confidentiality. The one-to-one interviews were also explained while the participant information sheets were distributed and explained, both within groups and on individual basis as the situations warranted. Some members who wanted more explanation volunteered to give the researcher their contact numbers and subsequent appointments were made, during which explanation and clarification were provided. The individuals who volunteered to participate were, therefore, checked to ensure that they met the inclusion criteria, and arrangements were made for the venues and dates appointments for the service users who volunteered to participate in focus group and one-to-one interviews. The administration of the participant information sheets and obtaining signatures for the consent forms were conducted before the respective interview sessions. The data collection exercise was carried out between the months of April and August 2016, in accordance with the timelines of this study.

Part III

Introduction

These concluding chapters comprise discussion of the findings of this study, including as it relates to the literature, the implications of the findings to mental health services, including policy, clinical and community settings, the limitations and future research opportunities presented by this study, and conclusion.

1| Discussion of Study Findings

1.1. Introduction

The results from the focus groups and one-to-one interviews indicate that there are varying degrees of LOC in the mental health experiences of the study participants. It was indicated that most of the responses from the participants were based on their experiences as it related to their mental health challenges, including some narration of their pre-mental illness experiences.

1.2. Stressors of Daily Living, Temporary LOC Internality

Some indications emerged suggesting that there were some elements of internality in the LOC of the participants before they started to experience mental health challenges which led to the illness experiences. It was also found that the admission, assessment, hospital treatment and discharge experiences gave indications of externality in the mental health LOC of the participants due to the experiences of the participants being characterised by a lack of control. It also corroborates with literature that mental health service users from A & C populations often experienced coercive pathways to entry to mental health services, a lack of control whilst in hospital, as well as negative post hospital experiences (Bhui & Bhugra, 2002; Keating et al, 2002; Wilson, 2011). However, the post hospital experiences expressed in this study are indicated to have been characterised by a combination of both internality and externality in their LOC. It is also interesting that the internality was expressed from the ambit of a perception of a sense of 'freedom' from the hospital experiences. It, therefore, suggests that the perceived freedom was temporal, as the participants also expressed a view of having limited control over their lives in addition to their perceived experience of freedom from being discharged from hospitals. It also indicates that the temporality of this feeling of freedom was expressed from the ambit of the absence of control (externality) which arose from a lack of freedom to make decisions or exert control over important issues affecting their lives. Most of the issues of concern expressed by the participants as having contributed to the externality in their LOC include a lack of control over housing, finances and medication. This also supports literature that many service users struggle with financial and housing challenges after their discharge from mental health hospitals, and struggle to cope with the challenges of side effects of medications (Schneider et al, 2010). It also suggests that the post discharge mental health LOC internality expressed was highly temporary and appear to be quickly cancelled out by a lack of control over other components of daily living which were considered highly important to the participants' sense of control over their lives, thereby leading to externality in their LOC.

It is also poignant to note that the findings of externality indicate that the participants were external in their LOC orientation in both general and mental health contexts, despite having been discharged from hospitals for a long period of time. It is, therefore, the view of the researcher that this study has presented a result to indicate that participants in this study are external in their LOC orientations in both general and mental health contexts, although the internality experienced in their mental health LOC was temporary in nature. The internality elements were observed in two main contexts – the period prior to what was expressed by most participants as 'breakdown' leading to mental illness, and period immediately post their hospital discharge experiences.

As discussed under the analysis section, the issues that contributed to LOC internality prior to the experiences and impacts of stressors that led to mental health challenges included the ability of the participants to exert control over their lives including being in control over their employment, relationship issues, identity issues, and financial issues. The LOC externality started to develop as soon as the participants started to experience challenges from racial discrimination, bullying, employment, and relationships. This also corroborates the literature that indicated that mental health challenges are often attributed to the impact of stressors such as relationship breakdown, employment stresses and alcohol/drug (McCabe & Priebe, 2004). Other factors in this finding corroborated by literature include a link between racism and mental ill health in ethnic minorities (McKenzie, 2008; Keating, 2012), and the impact of bullying on adult mental health including depression, anxiety and 'suicidality' (Takizawa et al, 2014: 171).

The externality in LOC found from the participants in this study has also identified the existence of a link between culture and LOC, which also corroborates the suggestion by literature that BME peoples who are collectivist are external in their LOC (Cheng et al, 2013). However, the LOC externality was found to be a product of perceived racism by the participants in both admission, hospital and post hospital experiences. This also corroborates literature assertion that ethnic minority service users experience racism with psychiatric services as explained under the literature review, including institutional racism (Sashidharan, 2001). It also includes the importance of family in decision making in general. However, in contrast to what obtains in literature, there appears to be a difference in LOC orientation in mental health context, as the A & C service users in this study were found to be internal in their mental health LOC in relation to discussing their challenges with family members. The factors that were perceived to have caused, contributed or played a role in the mental illness experiences of the study participants, the perception of the participants to the attitude of the mental health services and professionals, in particular the psychiatrists to the culture of the study participants, which combined with the perception of racism and racial discrimination.

Other issues found in this study include the fear of re-hospitalisation, the feeling of dependency on the state for livelihood and survival, the role of culture on the perception of control, the influence of perception of power on the responses of the participants to the services as well as their health seeking behaviours, as well as the perspectives of the study participants on how the mental health services and the community members could take actions to improve the LOC and, as a consequence, improve the experiences of the interviewed populations in mental health settings.

1.3. Making Decisions

The superordinate and accompanying subtopics around decision making found in this study indicates that three major factors influence decision making by the participants. This includes the influence of family and friends in relation to decisions on general issues, which corroborate the assertion by literature that BME groups belong to collectivist cultures and are external in their LOC (Cheng et al, 2013); a difference in approach to seeking support, advice or consultation in relation to decision making about mental health issues, and the role of spirituality and belief, including prayers and consultation with church leaders. The findings indicate that some elements of internality in LOC were expressed in relation to consulting family and friends, which corroborate literature's view that A & C peoples would avoid discussing their mental health challenges with family and friends (Keating, 2016; Mantovani et al, 2016). LOC externality in relation to the role of spirituality in decision making around mental health was also indicated in the findings, which also corroborates literature's assertion that members of A & C groups tend to seek support for psychological challenges from churches and faith leaders (Mantovani et al, 2016; Edge, 2013).

There is, however, a difference in the internal-external LOC orientation when the issues around making decisions regarding mental health arise. This is accompanied by internality in LOC, as the participants would generally not consult family members and friends when they need to decide on mental health issues. The external LOC element in this respect was demonstrated in consulting only people with experience of mental health challenges.

The findings in relation to the LOC of the A & C groups in this study in relation to decision making challenges the general notion in literature that people from BME backgrounds generally subscribe to externality in their decision making in general and in mental health settings. The flaw in this notion lies in the fact that it has not taken into account what has now been found in this study that there is an observed difference in approach by groups from A & C populations; that they mostly express differences in internality and externality in decision making in different contexts- general context and mental health context. This suggests that there now exists an addition to knowledge in this regard which lies in the finding that although there is some element of externality with regards to making decisions on general issues, externality in LOC appear to apply in a different degree to the A & C groups in relation to making decisions on issues around mental health challenges.

Therefore, the findings from this study further suggests that mental health service users from A & C populations are likely to express external LOC on general issues as they rely on family and friends, their religious leaders as well as value spirituality before making decisions. They nevertheless lean more towards internality in LOC when they face some challenges regarding their mental health. This is because they would not consult other people, especially family and friends for support or advice in making mental health related decisions. Conversely, as they are likely to consult people whom they have ascertained to have previous experience of the type of mental health challenges they were about to make decisions on, it suggests that their externality in this regard is based on their conscious sense of internality to seek out and rely on people with previous experiences of mental health challenges.

This finding regarding internality in relation to decision making by these sampled groups also seem to highlight the role played by stigma, lack of understanding, shame, fear of loss of privacy, fear of services and trust issues within the A & C groups, which, in turn, results in people facing mental health challenges making the decision to avoid discussing their challenges with their family members and friends (Keating et al, 2002; Keating, 2016). A nuanced consideration of the LOC internality found here suggests that it may be due to socio-cultural factors and stigma. This also corroborates assertion in literature that members of the A & C populations who experience mental health challenges avoid seeking help from family members due to stigma, including family rejection and becoming alienated from their communities (Mantovani et al, 2016). This has been described as "internalized 'self-stigma'" (Mantovani et al, 2016: 9). This further raises an issue around the likelihood that service users from these populations may not access support when they need it, and thereby contribute to lateness in receiving such support, as well as contribute to the entry to mental health services at crisis points (Keating, 2016). It suggests also that there is a possibility that they may not find people with experiences of mental health challenges to confide in and rely on their experiences to support them. It also raises issue around the level of trust and understanding within these populations, which may be contributory to the coercive pathways by A & C service users, especially considering that members of these groups are considered to be collectivist in culture and the role of family and friends are important in the collectivist societies.

The issue of reliance on spiritual beliefs in decision making as expressed in the topics of findings also suggests the existence of externality in LOC by this sample of A & C service users, as a result of the expressed reliance on spiritual beliefs, prayers and the consultation with church leaders. This finding also suggests that salient issues are being raised regarding the extent to which services need to pay attention to the spiritual beliefs of the service users from these populations in their interactions and engagement with them in mental health settings. It would suggest that there is a possibility that their decisions to engage or not to engage with services may be influenced by the spiritual beliefs; this, in turn, indicates that mental health services need to explore these beliefs alongside the service users from these groups in order to gain a better understanding of their motivation and how they can be supported.

1.4. Externality in LOC

The literature suggests that BME people are externally oriented in their LOC in both general and mental health contexts. The findings of this study from the results indicate that the A & C participants lean to both externality in their general LOC and mental health LOC. This suggests that as participants had expressed levels of control in decision making in different contexts as it relates to their mental health experiences, they had levels of internality and externality. This, in turn, suggests that the notion by literature that the BME populations are external in their LOC may not be entirely applicable to mental health service users from the A & C groups in mental health contexts.

The findings also suggest that certain factors which were indicated to have played a role in the LOC of participants in this study (such as perception of stigma and lack of experience of mental illness by family members indicated by the participants in this study as reasons for not discussing their mental health challenges with family members), may have been omitted or not considered in the literature. This, further, suggests that the generalisation by the literature that all groups of BME extraction tend to be external in mental health LOC may be flawed. The viewpoint of literature also seems to have not taken into consideration the contexts and specific differences of the subject groups that have been explored in this study. Such differences include historical, migration, socio-cultural issues as well as experiences of discrimination, racism and institutional racism that have been experienced in mental health services by the A & C groups (McKenzie & Bhui, 2007).

1.5. Phases of Internality and Externality

The findings suggest that the existence of several shifts in the mental health LOC of the participants were in correlation to the stages of their mental illness experiences.

As illustrated in Figure 3 (Driver of Phenomenon of Temporality in MHLOC in A & C mental health experiences), below, this includes the periods before their mental illness was triggered, the admission process, hospitalisation stages, the in-hospital experiences, discharge experiences and conditions that accompanied their discharge, and their experiences after discharge from hospital. These stages are characterised by different types of the Internal and External (I-E) conditions.

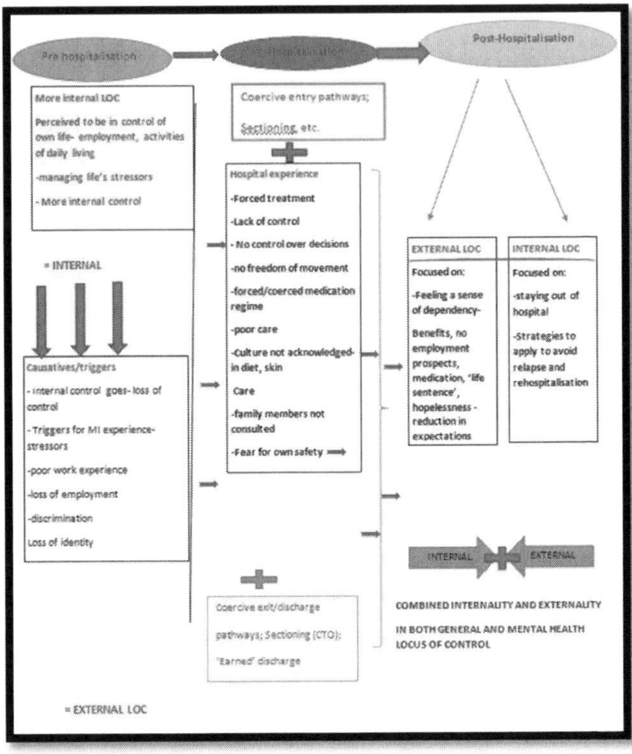

Figure 3: Driver of Phenomenon of Temporality in MHLOC in A & C Mental Health Experiences

Figure 3 (Driver of Phenomenon of Temporality in MHLOC in A & C mental health experiences), is an illustration of how the LOC is impacted by several stages of the mental health experiences of the A & C service users. It includes: the periods before mental illness was triggered (characterised by LOC internality), the admission process and hospitalisation stages, and the in-hospital experiences and discharge experiences and conditions that accompanied their discharge (characterised by externality in LOC); and the post-hospital experiences (characterised by a combination of LOC internality and externality)

These stages are explained further below:

1.5.1. The Period before and Immediate to Mental Illness

The results indicate that the participants' experiences were characterised by a commencement from a condition of a more internal orientation before the initial experience of mental illness leading to hospitalisation, which changes to externality during hospitalisation. As most participants expressed that prior to their experiences of stresses in their lives which led to trigger of mental illness, they perceived that they were in control of their lives. This state of internal LOC also seems to be short-lived (some elements of temporality), as they started to experience challenges to their wellbeing, due to factors including relationship breakdowns, stresses at work, questions regarding their identity, family issues, financial problems, perceived racial discrimination, drug and alcohol issues, etc. These factors seem to have combined to lead to externality, which, in turn, led to breakdown.

1.5.2. Hospitalisation

The experience of breakdown impacted by these earlier observed stressors has been found in this study to have been followed by the hospitalisation experience which was also characterised by externality due to the perceived lack of control expressed by most of the participants. This is mainly due to the opinion expressed that they were not involved in the decision made by people other than themselves to admit them to hospital for assessment and treatment. This externality continued as the assessment, treatment and hospital stay experiences were characterised by a perception a lack of control in decisions made on their behalf by the professionals in relation to medication, diagnosis, care, experience of coercion, experience of helplessness, perception of having to 'earn' discharge, perceived poor care due to mental health services ignoring their culture and other factors highlighted in the qualitative topics. This stage of hospitalisation is, therefore, characterised by a high degree of externality.

1.5.3. The Post Hospitalisation Period

It is subsequently characterised by two elements of externality and internality. The externality is characterised by factors highlighted by the interviewees, which include being discharged on coercive conditions including Community Treatment Orders, a feeling of dependence on the state for livelihood via social benefits, the constraints around employment prospects due to the impact of the mental illness experiences, a perception of stigma, a feeling of hopelessness and a reduction in expectations. It is also characterised by a perception of fear of possible relapse and rehospitalisation thereby leading to a repeat of the experiences, which, in turn, seem to perpetuate the sense of externality in LOC.

The internality element is characterised by the feeling of 'freedom', being in control by making decision to exert some control over own life after hospitalisation, which resulted from the expressed freedom from perceived incarceration that characterised their hospital experiences; and a determination to avoid re-hospitalisation. This internality has, however, been expressed as temporal, as the majority of the participants seem to indicate the 'freedom' expressed was only in the parlance of gaining freedom of movement resultant from physically discharged and leaving hospital; as they expressed that the internality changed to externality due to the factors enumerated earlier.

1.6. Contradictory Internality and Externality (?)- Indication of the Phenomenology of Temporality

The findings of seemingly contradictory status of internality and externality and the temporal movement between internality and externality in the locus of control of the participants in this study suggests the applicability of the phenomenon of temporality as postulated by Husserl (Brough & Blattner, 2006). Husserl's phenomenology of temporality has at its centre the role played by time in perception of experiences. This phenomenology which later influenced the works of Heidegger, Sartre, and Merleau-Ponty, refers to the notion that time plays an important role in 'intentional' consciousness, perception, and experiences (Brough & Blattner, 2006; Fuchs & Van Duppen, 2017). It also highlights the temporality of awareness or consciousness, and consequently the need to be aware

interventions by mental health services towards avoiding repetition of negative experiences for clients are likely to reduce the fear and anxiety of what is to come, which is an element of LOC externality (a fear of the future). Such interventions are, therefore, likely to increase the level of their internality in their mental health LOC.

Furthermore, as literature suggests that the level of internality in the LOC of mental health clients is a determining factor in their engagement with services (Treacy et al, 2015), it proposes also that focusing on such factors identified as likely to increase internality are also likely to impact on their position on the internal-external (I-E) spectrum.

In exploring Merleau-Ponty's views on temporality and subjectivity in the Phenomenology of perception, Aguiar de Sousa (2017) suggests that: "Whenever we perceive something, we are always originally directed to a future horizon. Thus, the present phase of perception is always surrounded by a double horizon, one side corresponding to the immediate past, the other to the immediate future" (Aguiar de Sousa (2017: 13). The paradox indicated in this phenomenon of temporality highlights the extent to which the participants navigate the trajectories of possible rehospitalisation due to a relapse, which indicates that there is a likelihood of a repeat of the cycle of internality to externality and back to internality in their MHLOC. It also further highlights the impact of expectations or fear of relapse and hospital readmission expressed by many of the participants in this study, which, in turn, impact on their perception of externality in LOC.

1.7. Collectivism

As indicated in earlier chapter in this thesis, including the literature review and the qualitative analysis sections, literature suggests that BME people are culturally collectivist (Cheng, et al, 2013). The findings of this study have indicated that the A & C people base their decisions on general issues of importance on the importance of their family members. It has also been indicated that the A & C people rely on the views, opinions and advice of their family members before they make decisions on important issues.

As placing importance on family members and their role in decision making are characteristics of collectivist cultures, it indicates that this finding from this study in this regard has corroborated the suggestion by literature on a general basis. However, this view cannot be claimed to be entirely generalizable to the A & C community when the issue around mental health comes into focus. It has been found that the importance these study populations placed on family members seem to be affected by their concerns regarding the responses of their family members to mental health challenges. As indicated in the findings of this study, the issue around stigma, fear, shame and family reputation seems to play a role in the way the people of A & C backgrounds relate to the importance of their family members when they experience mental health challenges.

The collectivism concept also appears to be observed by the participants in their expectations that their family members be involved by health professionals in their care experiences in mental health settings, which they, in turn, expressed was not forthcoming. The findings from this study, therefore, indicates that collectivism has been demonstrated in mental health contexts by this sample of African and Caribbean mental health service users, thereby confirming to a large extent the suggestions by literature, albeit with some reservations dictated by mental health stigma.

1.8. Summary- Discussion

This study has explored the participants' responses to the interview questions in relation to their perception of control of their lives. This exploration has thrown more light to the perceived reasons for the externality in their LOC- which has now been identified as due to a combination of factors including their own experiences of social stressors which led to mental health challenges and breakdown, issues related to assessment, hospital admission, treatment, discharge and after discharge stages of their experiences with mental health services, which were perceived to have been driven by experiences of racial discrimination and other social inequalities.

The study also enabled the 'world view' of the study participants to be explored, using the idiographic approach of the Interpretative Phenomenological Analysis (IPA). The researcher has also been able to rely on the participants' expression of their own perception from their own experiences to describe as well as interpret those expressions. This strategy has also enabled an in-depth and through level of finding into the likelihood of proffering solutions to the identified issues in the study, as most of the participants has also offered some suggestions as to how they perceived that the conditions and issues they expressed could be changed or improved. This indicates that the study has also achieved its aims and objectives as stipulated in the research questions.

The expressions of seemingly contradictory LOC within the context of the out of hospital experiences of the participants also raise the phenomenon of temporality in the LOC of the participants. As illustrated in Figure 3 (Driver of Phenomenon of Temporality in MHLOC in A & C mental health experiences), it highlights that different experiences impacted on their LOC, including the temporality in their internality and a sense of a continuation of externality in LOC in their post hospital experiences. It also raises the need to address the differences in their perception within the same contexts. It, therefore, seems to suggest that it is necessary to understand what factors may contribute to service users' externality with a view to reducing or addressing them in order to place them on a higher internality scale. These original findings which also point to temporality also present a novel start to a band of knowledge that is required into exploring the explanatory model for the experiences of this study population in mental health settings in the United Kingdom.

The foregoing assessment of the findings in relation to the stance of literature suggests that people of A & C backgrounds do subscribe to the collectivist cultures, as encompassed in the importance they place to members of their family on general issues, as well as it relates to their expected role in their mental health experiences. However, the findings indicate that the notion of externality in LOC claimed by literature for BME peoples (Cheng et al, 2013) may not be entirely generalizable in its applicability to A & C people, as they tend to exercise levels of both internality and externality as dictated by the stages and levels of their mental health experiences. In addition, a nuanced interpretation of the internality expressed by the participants in relation to not involving family members in mental health contexts suggests that stigma may play a role in such decisions, including fear of shame or becoming alienated from family members due to mental illness (Mantovani et al, 2016). It indicates that the internality in LOC must be viewed with caution, as the service user might have decided to keep the information to themselves and avoid seeking support, out of fear of stigma. The avoidance of services due to fear and stigma have been implicated to leading to the individual's condition getting worse, thereby leading to entry to services by coercive pathways (Keating, 2016). This indicates that this study presents an addition to the knowledge of the LOC status of the A & C groups as a subset of the BME groups in the United Kingdom. It also suggests that specific contexts of admission, hospital experiences and post discharge experiences need to be considered in order to place the LOC profiles of specific BME groups into consideration for exploration.

These findings present a distinctive contribution to knowledge, as there had been no known previous study which has explored these issues with mental health clients in general and African and African Caribbean groups in particular, in spite of the over representation of the study populations group in mental health settings in the United Kingdom. The concept of mental health LOC had hitherto not been analysed with these study populations (African and Caribbean service users) through the application of an in-depth method of a combination of one-to-one and focus group interviews with the use of semi structured interview questions. This analysis has also highlighted the role of family, identity, perception of levels of control in relation to stages of the mental illness course, differences in decision making between everyday important matters in comparison to mental health issues, the importance of culture and the views of the participants in relation to the mental health services attitude to their culture and consequently their experience with and response to services.

2| Implications of and Recommendations from Research Findings for A & C Mental Health

The findings from this study suggest the following implications for mental health in both clinical and community settings, and what needs to be considered and actioned by mental health services and policy makers as it relates to mental health service users from A & C populations. This is more poignant because public authorities have acknowledged that the challenges regarding the mental health profiles of the BME populations are complex. It has, indeed, been stated in one of recent CQC reports in respect of overrepresentation of BME groups in the use of MHA detentions that "the reasons why the MHA is used more in some Black and minority ethnic (BME) groups are complex and not well understood (CQC, 2016: 19). This indicates that the findings in this study have the potential to add a greater level of understanding of actions that need to be taken to address the challenges.

- Culture appears to play a role in the externality found in the LOC of the sampled population in their experience of mental health and services. This includes the demonstration of several characteristics of collectivism which comprises the importance placed on family members in decision making and expectations in healthcare contexts. There was, however, a perception that this aspect of their lives has not been acknowledged by services and professionals, including a lack of inclusion of their family members in their health care. LOC externality can be reduced, and internality increased if the family members are included in decisions and the healthcare process. This finding in this study regarding importance placed by the sampled population on their family members seem to confirm the position in a recent study on interventions which involved family members of groups of African Caribbean backgrounds with diagnosis of schizophrenia, that "Family intervention is one approach which may improve African-Caribbean clients' engagement with mainstream services, encourage more timely access to care (via less coercive pathways) and improve risk management; thereby enabling better care experiences and outcomes" (Edge, 2011: 2-3). This suggests that clinicians need to include family members in their engagement with this population in all mental health settings for positive outcomes.

- The literature also suggests that groups of collectivist cultures who are in the minority in a society are likely to "accept" dominant power as a given/norm and may not protest its dominance (Cheng et al, 2013). This would indicate that externality in LOC found in this study could be a demonstration of a response of groups of collectivist cultural persuasion to the perceived dominant power exerted by services. It would suggest therefore that the link between collectivism and externality is applicable to groups of A & C population. It suggests also that health professionals need to consider addressing the externality by promoting internality (Norman et al, 1998). They also need to acknowledge and address the perception of the dominance of the power of services in the clients-services engagement by increasing the active participation, and adopting the needs, views and opinions of the A & C client in the healthcare process, thereby increasing their sense of control. It also means that services must encourage active participation of the clients from the A & C groups in decision making, listen and take on board their views, as well as focus on their expressed needs.
- Affiliated to this is the involvement of family members, significant others and friends in the health care process, as expressed by the participants. This means that services must acknowledge the need for the triangle of care to be observed in both clinical and community settings. This should be based

on the expressed need of the clients. Efforts should also be made by services to know the members of the family of their clients and those who are interested and want to play an active role in their care and include them in the process. There is also a strong need for therapeutic communication to be promoted among the health professionals and the clients and family members (Bhui et al, 2013).

- It has been posited that externality in LOC could also support health professionals in their interventions related to improving active participation and health promotion related behaviour (Buhagiar, et al, 2011). This would suggest that there are some positive elements to LOC externality, as 'it places healthcare professionals in a very favourable position to exert their influence by means of health promotion and active therapeutic interventions that reduce modifiable risk factors for physical disease and improve outcomes' (Buhagiar, et al, 2011:1). It also suggests that professionals can provide some clinical and community support by applying their LOC externality to support A & C clients in their recovery at the initial stages whilst applying some interventions to increase their LOC internality. However, considering the challenges of perceived inequality, racism and discrimination expressed by participants in this study, as corroborated by the literature as implicated in negatively impacting help-seeking in this population (Mantovani et al, 2016), the success of this approach will be dependent on the level of genuine trust between the service user and the professional.
- Spirituality, including, beliefs in God, prayers and consultation with spiritual leaders including church leaders appear to play a role in the level of externality in the LOC of the sampled population. It also appears to impact on their decision making and help-seeking attitudes in relation to mental health. Literature has indicated that spirituality plays an important role in help-seeking behaviours of A & C peoples in relation to

mental health, including the socio-cultural role of faith-based organisations, pastors, spiritual leaders and Black Majority Churches (Mantovani et al, 2016; Edge, 2013). It has also been posited that A & C groups rate the support from churches, pastors and other spiritual leaders highly when they experience mental health challenges. However, the response of such leaders may not necessarily be positive, as psychological challenges may be perceived by those leaders as signs of unbelief, demonic or spiritual weakness, thereby tending to promote stigma in the A & C communities (Mantovani et al, 2016). The LOC externality indicated here in relation to spirituality and beliefs appears to be a product of socio-cultural factors which need to be considered by the health professional.

- It suggests that interventions by health professionals need to inculcate the spiritual beliefs of this population as it relates to their mental health experiences. This includes listening to them to find out how their belief system plays a role in their mental health and their responses, and how they can be supported to explore their faith in ways that can complement the interventions to achieve positive outcomes. This requires an acknowledgement of spirituality by the professionals as a complementary psycho-socio-cultural factor to the medical model, rather than a conflicting concept, as this has been raised as a challenging issue with the medical model (Edge, 2013). It also highlights a need for training in social work, nursing and other health care practices, especially given their roles as AMHPs to acknowledge spirituality and take it into account in their dealings with A & C service users. Continuous Professional Development approaches also need to inculcate the need for practitioners to balance service user and community perspectives respectively in their practices as it relates to A & C service users.

- Most participants expressed a sense of powerlessness, fear, and inadequacy in their experiences with services, which is attributed to the perception that their opinions, views, and responses are not acknowledged in their engagement with services. Fear in psychiatric services has been raised in literature in relation to the experiences of A & C service users with mental health services (Keating et al, 2002). The fear of forced readmissions, a lack of input into the medication regime and inadequate support after discharge appear to be high on the concerns. It suggests that LOC externality can be reduced by encouraging active participation of this population in the healthcare process and by giving them a sense of control in their engagement with services.
- Several cultural issues emanated as explanatory for the LOC externality by the participants; this includes the view regarding culturally specific diets, lack of support for skin and hair care, and identity focused activities during hospital admissions. These issues are also perceived to impact on their mental health outcomes. It suggests that interventions in clinical settings need to focus on the cultural needs of this population with regard to skin, hair care and culturally specific diets including A & C meals as has been articulated by the participants in this study. Making an inquiry and providing for the clients' culturally specific needs as opposed to making provisions to them based on the general population will be a better approach and increase internality in LOC.
- A perceived inadequacy of post-discharge support appears to exert influence on the LOC of the sampled population. This includes inadequate support for exploring employment prospects, inadequate housing and support networks in the community. These have also been expressed in the parlance of isolation, a lack of hope for the future, and poor employment

prospects thereby increasing externality. It suggests that post-hospital interventions and support need to be targeted at raising a sense of hope for the future, and raising self-confidence, self-esteem and a sense of empowerment for the client by addressing their economic needs and reduce isolation. Providing adequate housing and support to explore employment prospects will go a long way in increasing internality and promote engagement with health services in this population.

- Pressure from government agencies to seek employment has been highlighted by participants. This has been described as inconsiderate as it affects their LOC and promotes relapses. Government agencies should promote active support to avoid clients being pressured into employment when they did not feel mentally and socially stable.
- Part of the inadequacy of post-hospital support highlighted by the participants was also in relation to venues for social activities and places where they can access support in the community. As many participants articulated that the impact of medication and side effects affected their ability to explore employment prospects, they need places where they can go to socialise and participate in activities that are not related to employment, thereby addressing isolation and promote their wellbeing. It has been asserted that health can be improved with the availability of activities in community settings. This includes "Almost anything that brings groups together in a variety of ways such as religious groups, choirs, yoga classes, schools, youth and community centres have the potential to enhance health" (Edge & West, 2011: 21). This suggests that the health care providers must seek ways to provide venues where groups of A & C backgrounds with experience of mental health challenges can go and meet other groups in the community to participate in health-promoting activities. The professionals also need to seek out places for such activities

available in the community for their clients, thereby improving their sense of confidence and control in their health and wellbeing.

- This is closely related to funding, as services and governments need to fund culturally focused centred where A & C groups can attend and participate in activities to raise their LOC, and where peer support can be encouraged. Health awareness and promotional activities can also be organised for these groups in those centres.
- The view regarding culture appears to have an impact on the LOC externality level of the population in their engagement with services and health professionals, especially the psychiatrist. The majority of the participants' view regarding the historical attitude of A & C peoples to the health professionals (that the latter have superior knowledge and unquestionable authority), and the perception of inferiority of A & C culture, education and skills to the (predominantly White) professionals, which are attributed to a combination of historical oriented racism, were expressed as reasons for their feeling of a lack of confidence and sense of control in engagement with services.
    - On the other hand, the perception that health professionals have an inferior view of the A & C cultures, coupled with the perception that the professionals tend to ignore cultural issues also appear to play a role in the LOC externality, thereby leading to a lack of motivation to exert control in their engagement with services. It suggests that raising awareness and increasing training of the professionals regarding African and Caribbean culture may help in reducing the expressed unsatisfactory experiences. It also corroborates suggestion from literature for a need for cultural competency of the health professionals (Bhui & O'Hara, 2014).

- It also suggests that further education of the A & C service users regarding equality of cultures, the responsibility of services and professionals, and their rights as service users could raise their awareness, confidence and LOC in their engagement with services and professionals. This can be addressed by both services and charity organisations.
- As expressed by most of the participants, services and policymakers need to consider increasing the staff strength of their senior and decision-making echelons with professionals from A & C populations. They also need to provide career advancement and training opportunities for professionals from these groups, in order to enable the act as role models for the service users from A & C groups. They also suggested that this will ensure that professionals with an understanding of the historical and socio-cultural differences and needs of the A & C groups are embedded in the service provisions and mental health support. This may also reduce the externality which arose from the perception that the staffing is not representative of the clientele in respect of ethnicity and racial differences.
- Health professionals from the mainstream and other backgrounds should also demonstrate an interest in the culture of their clients, familiarise themselves with them and genuinely acknowledge their cultural needs by developing their relationship with them.
- The importance of culture in diets and health has also been highlighted by the participants, thereby suggesting that a review of the food served to service users from A & C populations, and other BME groups in hospital settings is overdue, with a view to seeking ways to provide culturally focussed meals to this category of clients.
- The seemingly contradictory status of both internality and externality in LOC in the post-discharge experiences of most of the participants is a major finding in this study. This is

highlighted in the shift between a feeling of a sense of control from perceived sense of freedom which arose from being discharged from hospital (internality of LOC), to a feeling of a lack of control due to perceived sense of inability to influence decisions or lack of control over their post-discharge care, which also led to the perception that they had to 'fight' to receive the care they needed (LOC externality).

- Considering that mental health service users from A & C populations continue to express powerlessness and a lack of involvement in decisions relating to their care, it suggests that previous initiatives over the years which focused on the challenges of BME mental health, including the *Delivering Race Equality* (DRE) cited in the literature review of this study (Williams et al, 2006; Crisp et al, 2016), has had little impact on the experiences of A & C service users. It also indicates that the results from the *Count Me In* census of 2010 (Care Quality Commission, 2011), has not impacted positively on the experiences of the A & C service users. It means that services, the government and policymakers need to revisit these reports and recommendations from these initiatives, including the need to incorporate the perspectives of service users and family members.
- As issues of racism, discrimination, and a lack of attention to ethnicity and cultural needs have also been expressed by participants in this study, it highlights a lack of impact of the government's mental health policy initiatives aimed at promoting equality in mental health access and experiences as it relates to BME communities. It also raises the need for policymakers to revisit the previous policies with a view to identifying and eliminating the challenges to their implementation.
- Although the Care Act (2014) has provisions for personalised care, the perception of a 'one cap fits all' approach by services expressed by participants in this study suggests that

depersonalisation was experienced by them. Services, therefore, need to pay particular attention to the opportunities the Care Act (2014) it offers for more personalised care which focuses on the needs of the service user, including the role of local authorities working in conjunction with mental health services in the provision of post-hospital care, with their personal involvement in decision making (DoH, 2014).

- The government has commenced an independent review of the Mental Health Act, which has been indicated to include investigating reasons behind disproportionate detention rates of Black, Asian and minority ethnic people under the act (DoH, 2017). There is a need for the review to also pay particular attention to the minimal result of previous policy initiatives, and incorporate other options that could be available, including processes that services and professionals can use to build trust between services and service users from the A & C groups and family members.
- The government and services should also promote and fund co-production of services in the communities, and service user involvement in the creation of services.
- In the light of the limited impact of policy initiatives, the government, policymakers, and services need to pay particular attention to various research evidence that has suggested the need for greater service user involvement, funding of community groups, and the co-production of services.
- As indicated earlier in the literature review, since the end of the *DRE*, and the final report on the *Count me in* census (Crisp et al, 2016), there has been no specific government policy which directly addresses issues of racism and racial inequality in services as it relates to BME populations' over-representation in mental health settings. This includes the recent government document titled "Achieving Better Access to Mental Health Services by 2020" (DoH, 2014: 18). It

suggests that the discourses relating to racial inequality in mental health has gone to the back burner while racial discourses in relation to mental health outcomes are not only no longer current topics but has become a difficult topic to discuss in the British society (Mulholland, 2017). However, recent indications still highlight that A & C and other BME peoples are still currently over-represented in psychiatric services (McManus et al, 2016). This suggests that discourses around racism and racial discrimination in psychiatric services should no longer be ignored, but need to resume and be promoted, as it has been posited that suggesting cultural competence towards improving minority ethnic mental health "locate the issue(s) at an individual level and ignore the deleterious consequences of racism, racial inequality, and structural disadvantage" (Keating, 2016: 176).

- The findings from this study also raise implications for health and social care professionals, particularly the role of the social workers and psychiatric nurses as Approved Mental Health Practitioners (AMHP). It suggests that professionals need to not only be kept abreast of the ethnicity and cultures of A & C peoples who may be indicated to be experiencing mental health challenges in their assessment and intervention roles in the communities. Professionals also need to be continually trained as an integral part of their Continuous Professional Development on culturally sensitive issues that relate to A & C service users they care for in their roles. Social work, nurses and other healthcare students should also be exposed to knowledge and information regarding racial, cultural and historical factors that impact on health and wellbeing in the various communities. This is because the AMHPs are more likely to be involved in the more controlling aspects of care in community contexts, including the processes of 'sectioning' under the Sections 2 and 3 of the Mental Health Act, as well as the administration of the provisions of Community Treatment Orders (CTOs). It also raises the need to balance service user and community perspectives, respectively, including the notions of equilibrium between respecting the human rights of the service user and the need to adhere to public safety requirements under the Mental Health Act. It also suggests that AMHPs must take a holistic view of all their clients as well as consider ethnicity and cultural factors in their interactions with A & C peoples and their decision-making processes. They must also base their judgements on the provisions of Section 17 of the Mental Health Act relating to post-hospital experiences of the service user and the Care Act (2014), how they impact on their ethnicity and cultural needs, as well as are kept up to date with current regulations relating to the rights of the service users.

- The findings in this study relating to racism and inequality affecting A & C service users also highlights the importance of the role of social work, which has been described as an 'intersection of multidisciplinary and interagency practice of mental health' (Keating, 2016: 180). It suggests that as social work is by nature expected to advocate and promote social justice, it is challenged to pay particular attention to the impact of the various issues which contribute to externality of the LOC of the service user can be addressed by addressing such perceptions in their interaction with the clients. This includes building trust, understanding and adopting a holistic and person-centred approach to the clients, bearing in mind the fluidity of identities. It has also been suggested that social work is positioned to be mindful of how race and mental health intersect, and that, 'mental health social workers can promote an understanding of the complexities of racialized identities and how social structures as well as anti-Black Sanism affect the conditions of daily living for racialized groups' (Keating, 2016: 180).

2.1. Author's Thoughts - The Role of Reflexivity on Study

Reflexivity has been described as a process by which the researcher continuously engages in self-reflection into awareness about their actions, feelings and views (Darawsheh, 2014; Anderson 2008). It has also been asserted that rigour can be accomplished when a researcher reflects on how factors such as "their cultural background; thoughts; actions; emotions; assumptions; and unconscious responses" might impact the process and findings of a study (Darawsheh, 2014: 563). These factors were deliberately considered by the researcher in the course of this study in order to ensure that reflexivity was adhered to.

In the first place, the researcher went into conducting this study involving Black participants with some misgivings. This include concerns regarding the likely impact of the researcher being a Black man, a psychiatric nurse, and a Black psychiatric nurse might have on the response to an invitation to participate, the course of participation, and the ultimate outcome of the study. Concern was also internalised by the researcher about how the status of someone with these characteristics of a Black male, psychiatrist nurse, a Black psychiatric nurse, who was conducting a research into their 'own' community might affect how the potential participants might respond to an invitation to participate in the study and their willingness to do so (Egharevba, 2001). In addition, it was a concern as to how the participants would see the researcher in view of these factors. This has been referred to as 'placing', which has been defined as 'The ways in which the personal characteristics of the researcher and the researched such as, but not exclusively, class, 'race'/ethnicity, and gender, assist the researched in locating the researcher within wider social structures (and vice versa) (Mirza) (1998: 84–85). These thoughts, therefore, pervaded the mind of the researcher in the course of approaching the organisations and service users, as well as throughout the data collection process.

However, the concerns regarding response to invitation to participate was completely alleviated in the course of contact with charity organisations through whom access to the service users were gained, as the responses were highly positive. Indeed, the responses seemed to indicate that although there were some element of ambivalence expressed by some of the service users to the fact that another researcher was making a request for participation in a study involving mental health service users, there seemed to have been a genuine willingness by the majority of A & C service users to participate in the study. This information was obtained from the coordinators of the two charity organisations involved in the recruitment, who also advised that the service users were already used to experiences of requests for participation in studies.

The researcher, however, found that some element of curiosity was also expressed by the service users from A & C community, and most of the potential participants expressed interest in the study. The researcher wondered if this curiosity was perhaps because it was being conducted by a Black male. It was also found that the researcher's status as a psychiatric nurse was not seen as a threatening factor for most of the participants.

Another concern internalised by the researcher was in relation to a consideration of the information and prior knowledge and pre-existing views of the researcher around inequality in mental health outcomes and over representation of the service users of the A & C community as indicated in the research interest section earlier in this report, and the extent to which such pre-existing views were likely to impact the study.

It was, therefore, very important to the researcher that reflexivity be consciously applied during this study by paying particular attention to researcher's subjectivity and achieving rigour which are necessary for the generation of credible findings, throughout the study process (Darawsheh, 2014). This was also based on the intention to ensure that attention was paid to issues such as the recruitment criteria, sampling techniques and interview questions. It was also necessary to ensure that the researcher's profession as a mental health nurse did not constitute a bias in the interviews, as the participants were given the opportunity to air their views and share their experiences. The use of semi structure questions and the pilot process were also aimed at ensuring that the questions were realistic and easily understood without being intrusive (Thabane et al, 2010). It was also consciously considered that the social status of the researcher as a member of the A & C community, coupled with the researcher's views on the issues being explored could have influenced the design of the interview schedule and focus group guide, the questioning technique applied and the analysis of data.

The concern regarding interview questions were dealt with by the support of the researcher's supervisor to ensure that the questions were objectively designed. This was also followed up by a pilot of the questions, as reported earlier, in order to eliminate bias. Efforts were also made in the interview techniques applied to ensure that the participants did not feel pressured to air their views in the use of prompts in the interview schedule and focus group guide, and they were informed that they were free to choose not to respond to any of the questions if they did not feel comfortable to do so.

It was also necessary to ensure that the topics that emerged in the analysis were clearly examined to capture participants' views in the interpretation. However, as discussed under limitation of findings in the final section of this report, the researcher was mindful of unconscious bias that could have emanated from his role as an interviewer, and the possibility that the interviewees' responses to some questions might have been influenced by what the participants perceived that the researcher wanted to hear (Alshenqeeti, 2014), especially given that the participants were informed of the researcher's profession as a psychiatric nurse. The researcher had offered assurance of anonymity and confidentiality to the participants that the interview was within their control and that they were free to express their views. This assurance was also repeated at the start of each on-to-one interview and focus group sessions.

The researcher's experience from this study has highlighted how the interpretation of individual's interactions within their social world in the environment they live in, and their experiences with services, can impact on their own interpretation of reality and their responses to such reality. The researcher has been impressed by the need to be aware of the importance of keeping an open mind to service users' experiences and subject every case to scrutiny. This is in the light of the various factors that can act as limitations, stressors and opportunities towards the client's wellbeing, particularly in view of the impact of the medical model, which pays minimal attention to the social and personal situations of the service user.

Although Fade (2004), highlighted phenomenologists view that the researcher need to acknowledge their own beliefs, opinions and pre-suppositions, it is the view of the researcher from a reflection on the experience from this study that the majority of the participants in this study were able to express their opinions in spite of knowing that their views might not have been shared by the researcher as a mental health professional, albeit a Black male who is also a member of the community. This indicates that the researcher's bias might have had little effect on the ability of the participants as service users to express their opinions without fear or pressure. It is also a considered view of the researcher that a negative influence of researcher power was not noticeable in the course of this study, as the participants were observed to feel comfortable to express their views without feeling coerced or intimidated. This was demonstrated in the fluidity of the discussions in the focus group settings, and the positive feedback received during the debrief sessions for both one-to-one interviews and focus groups, as the majority also expressed they found the exercise a good and rewarding experience, as they were able to also make suggestions, as their opinions had not been sought in the past in the manner the interviews were conducted.

The researcher also found that being a Black male and a health professional who is a researcher might have had a positive impact on the participants' response to the questions, as it may have elicited some level of trust or confidence to express their views to someone from their own community whom they share similar characteristics with. This suggests a confirmation of the view that it is a natural response to lean towards people with whom one has similar characteristics such as culture and appearance (Darawsheh, 2014). This suggests that rather than being a negative, the researcher's status as a Black male might have had a positive impact on the participation and the level at which views were expressed by the participants in the study.

From the researcher's experience, clinical settings are characterised by highly busy environments and schedules which do not necessarily offer opportunity for adequate interactions between professionals and service users to discuss their experiences and promote therapeutic engagements. It is, therefore, felt that this study has provided an opportunity to gain a greater insight into the service users' experiences and views. It has also disabused previous opinions of the researcher regarding the limitation of the role of the health professionals, and the need to pay more attention to the perception of the service users in relation to their social, cultural and personal circumstances, in both clinical and community settings, as it has now been highlighted from the findings that service users from A & C community do not feel that their opinions matter in the scheme of things in their experiences with services. It indicates also that professionals can do a lot to impact more positively on the wellbeing of the service user by listening more to and considering how the issues of collectivism in relation to relationship with family members can impact on their LOC and prevent them from seeking help.

The reflection on the findings in this study and the researcher's pre-existing views as a mental health practitioner in relation to the conflict between caring for service users and limiting their liberty suggests that the practitioners also need to take responsibility for the likely impact of control in mental health, with a view to supporting the client to minimise the negative impact of the coercive practices indicated in this report on their wellbeing. It also indicates that understanding of the ethnicity and cultures of A & C service users by mental health services, as well as practicing sensitivity that could help to change their LOC externality is not the only factor, neither can it be achieved by only a few practitioners but must be policy and practice-driven, with concerted efforts by all echelons of practice. Other socio-cultural factors such as institutional racism, societal racism, stigma and economic factors also need to be considered in a holistic approach to supporting individual service users.

This study has also addressed the researcher's curiosity to discover explanation for the over representation of A & C peoples in mental health settings in the UK, as the service user perspectives in this study has shed more light on the need to reflect on the intricacies involved in the mental health experiences of A & C service users in a racialised society. It has also impressed it on the researcher that the A & C and BME mental health profiles in the UK cannot be assessed in isolation but must be within the discourse of ethnicity, 'race' and culture, including historical considerations.

The researcher also found the status of a Black mental health practitioner being involved in conducting interviews with Black service users as an opportunity as opposed to having a negative impact. This is because BME groups have fallen within the contested notion of 'hard to reach' (Flanagan & Hancock, 2010; Garland et al, 2006). It is also considered that the Black status of the researcher offers a positive contrast to what has been criticised in cross-cultural research as 'White researchers studying minority issues' (Mio &Iwamasa, 1993: 202). It has also been observed that white researchers conducting research with BME research participants presents ethical and methodological issues (Edwards, 1996; Westwood & Allan, 2015), including those that particularly relate to power and privilege (Westwood & Allan, 2015; Muhammed et al, 2014). Indeed, it has been highlighted that questions have arisen as to 'whether non-members of marginalised communities could or should conduct research with members of those communities (Carling et al., 2013)'. (Westwood and Allan, 2015: 641).

The 'placing' element also appears to have resulted in a positive response by the service users in this study. However the researcher felt that some element of trust had to be established between the service users and the researcher to the extent that they felt comfortable enough to express their views, considering the role of the researcher as a health practitioner, which could have made the respondents feel that the researcher was an agent of the services from which they considered that they had been at the receiving end of coercive practices. In the light of this the researcher feels that the service users were more comfortable to speak with the researcher on sensitive issues and share their experiences, as they would have felt that they shared some commonality with the researcher as an individual from A & C background.

It is also the view of the researcher that the participants shared their views, experiences, opinions and suggestions in this study at such a depth that they would not have likely shared which a researcher who is not from the A & C community. This indicates a corroboration with the observation that similarity in identity, gender and experiences 'can create a shared empathy and a shared understanding between the respondents and the researcher in which trust and rapport can encourage respondents to open up and discuss their personal experiences (Bhopal, 2010: 188), which must have played a role in this study. In contrast, it has also been posited that in research with marginalised groups, 'it is widely accepted that ethnic and/or cultural differences in the backgrounds of researchers and research participants shape the research process (Culley, et al., 2007).' (Westwood & Allan, 2015: 641).

A final reflectivity point lies in the researcher's motivation in conducting this study, which includes an awareness of the over representation of the BME groups as service users in mental health settings, the challenges regarding racism and other social inequalities in a racialized society, and a desire to decipher answers towards addressing the challenges. However, the researcher made a conscious effort to ensure that the motivation did not impact on the recruitment, data collection, analysis processes, and that this report represents a balanced view of the findings. This is without pretending or hiding the fact that as a Black individual living in the same racialised society as the service users who are the respondents in this study, one naturally has strong feelings about the challenges, particularly the impact of social inequalities on the health and wellbeing of Black people in the UK.

The researcher has found it almost impossible to ignore the fact that the majority of A & C and BME peoples in the United Kingdom are exposed to negative experiences on several issues which impact on their activities of daily living (including unemployment, racism, prejudice, identity, and clash of cultures) at some times in their lives.

These negative experiences in a racialized society have a high potential to impact of their mental health and wellbeing, as they do not only form the basis of mental health challenges but tend to exacerbate mental illness. The researcher also reflected (with trepidation) on the negative issues raised from the experiences of the participants in this study with services and wonder if such could also happen to the researcher in the unlikely event of experiencing mental health challenges. It was, therefore, important to the researcher that the issues raised in this report are not only presented in a balanced way in accordance with the requirements of research rigour, but to also ensure that they are given the needed profile-raising to enable health practitioners, government and policy makers to take notice and necessary action towards improving the negative conditions. Overall, this exercise has opportuned the researcher to not only self-scrutinise and pay attention to the several issues including gender, identity, experience (Bhopal, 2010), culture, ethnicity, power, profession, and own views in relation to the researcher and participants' relationships (Bhopal, 2010), but also highlighted the importance of ensuring that rigour was observed in the entire research process with the support of the supervisor.

2.2. Conclusion - Implications and Recommendations

This study has provided an opportunity to unearth new sets of knowledge into the challenges of the mental health experiences of A & C service users. As the first study into assessing culture and LOC as a possible instructive model for the over-representation of A & C groups in mental health settings in England and the United Kingdom, this study has harnessed the benefits qualitative tools to achieve its aims and objectives via the research questions. It is also the first known attempt at applying a combination of one-to-one and focus group approaches to evaluate the LOC of A & C mental health service users; it has also resulted in delving into the perspectives of the target mental health clients in their perception of control in relation to various stages of their mental health experiences and the impact of their cultures.

The findings in this study underline the influence of history, migration, ethnicity, race and cultures in the perception of control of the A & C groups in their experiences of mental health services, including their understanding regarding causative factors of illness, their hospitalisation, treatment, and their after-discharge experiences. It is also argued that although the findings from this study corroborate the notion of collectivism in BME groups, it, however, challenges the general notion that groups of BME backgrounds lean to externality; as it has been suggested by the findings that this notion may not be entirely generalizable to the A & C groups in mental health context. This is due to observed varying degrees of differences and levels of internality and externality in the various stages of their mental health experiences.

This study has also presented evidence that demonstrates the existence of underlying factors that are responsible for differences in LOC between hospitalisation and discharge stages for A & C mental health service clients. These identified differences and the underlying factors could not have emanated from the use of quantitative methods such as questionnaires. This includes the role and importance of family members in mental health settings, the impact of historical and cultural attitudes of previous generations on the perception of control and attitude of present-day clients to the health professionals, especially the psychiatrists. This is a demonstration of the benefits of collecting data via a combination of focus groups and one-to-one interviews (Lambert & Loiselle, 2008). Other observed issues include the role played by the study participants' perception of control, power, coercion as well as the experiences of unsatisfactory care expressed by them, which led to a feeling of powerlessness and fear of readmission. The suggestions articulated towards the improvement of the services received by A & C groups in mental health contexts, including the professionals, the community and the approaches to the clients could also not have been accessed by relying on quantitative methods alone.

Furthermore, the interplay of culture, ethnicity and historical issues around race cannot be treated in isolation or ignored when the experiences of the A & C clients in their mental health challenges are being considered by policymakers and health professionals. Their view regarding the exercise of power, control and coercion by services should also not be ignored by the health professionals in their engagement with the A & C community. Efforts also need to be made by the professionals to demonstrate interest in the culture of the groups they serve, especially as it affects their views of mental health, issues regarding their perspective on family members' involvement in their mental health and support, the role of friends and other supporters as well as specific cultural needs.

This includes the need for health professionals to consider cultural issues in their assessment, treatment and other areas of their engagement with groups of A & C cultures in mental health settings. Addressing the socio-cultural issues that are not only causative but contributory to the illness experience is also of paramount importance.

The future health care system must aim to conduct interventions that could increase the internality of LOC of the mental health service users they serve from the A & C populations, promote their sense of control in the health care experiences by according them and their family members their right rather than privilege to be active decision makers in their healthcare and the processes that accompany their experiences. The high level of inadequacy of support with regards to housing, review of medication, employment and engagement of positive activities also need to be addressed for groups of A & C backgrounds after their discharge from hospitals, as these have been found to promote externality in their LOC. Provisions also need to be made by services for adequate cultural-specific support in the community settings whereby clients can be provided with opportunities to explore their potentials, especially after long periods of hospitalisation.

In conclusion, as has been posited by literature that LOC is a highly integral part of an active engagement with the healthcare process. The role played by the cultural paradigm of collectivism in mental health stigma has also been highlighted to impact on the LOC of the A & C service users, including self-imposed isolation. It is hereby argued that it is by considering the issues highlighted in the findings of this study and required specific actions taken by policymakers and the health professionals that the internality in the LOC of service users of A & C backgrounds can be promoted and empower them to take ownership of their health and wellbeing. This also has the potential to play a role in reducing the over-representation of A & C groups in mental health settings, as well as improve the challenges of BME mental health in general.

2.3. Implication for Other Minority Cultures? -Towards a Solution-Driven Bio Psycho Socio-Cultural Model

The various issues identified in the foregoing study highlights the importance of sensitivity to cultures, with particular focus on the role of collectivism in several minority cultures. In line with *'developmental model of intercultural sensitivity'* posited by Bennet, (1993), there appears to be a desirability for health and social care services to demonstrate the following understanding and actions in the engagement with clients, patients, consumers, or service users from ethnic cultures worldwide:

- Given that all mental health legislations are originally based on individualist orientation in developed countries, the various services and mental health practitioners need to recognise that peoples of culture who migrated or are descendants or migrants into these countries as well as indigenous peoples (including Canada and Australia) largely come from a collectivist persuasion. This suggests that the legislations (Mental Health Acts and their respective guidelines), and attendant practices deserve to be revisited if they are to meet the needs and expectations of peoples of collectivist society, rather than the current one cap fits all approach. This requires a thorough understanding of the phenomena on the part of the practitioners and policy makers.
- A recognition that people of collectivist cultures and the attendant experiences of historical and institutional racism, discrimination, the intersection of fear, power, control,

mistrust and the medical model (in contrast with a model that also encompasses the psychological, social and cultural aspects of the individual), and the attendant feeling of helplessness and hopelessness, all combine to promote poor response, engagement and the inability of the individual to take ownership and control of their mental health, along with other negative results. This seems to suggest a reason for the current situation as demonstrated in observed poor positive response of many peoples of culture with the Mental Health Services in developed countries. Services, therefore, need to be tailored to managing this orientation with a view to achieving a change in this orientation to internal LOC, which would impact positively on their response to the services and practitioners.

- An understanding that the ethnic community members (indigenous or of migrant backgrounds) are influenced by their cultural backgrounds, it suggests that there is a need to explore the respective cultures and how they impact on mental health challenges and presentations. One important aspect of this is the role of mental health stigma in ethnic cultures, the need for professionals to keep abreast of this, raise awareness and support family members to manage it for successful outcomes for the individual, the whole family and community.
- It has also been highlighted that individuals from collectivist cultures are more subject to external sources of influence, such as their family and friends than peoples from individualist persuasion and tend to accept the control from these sources as having a significant influence on themselves. This implies that these service users would value input from their family and friends in their experience of mental health issues, and therefore suggests that health professionals and mental health services in general need to include and involve the input of family members and carers in all the stages of the intervention

process for a successful outcome. This has, unfortunately, not been the practice in many developed countries including the United Kingdom, Canada, and Australia, until recently. This also suggests that highly culturally sensitive intervention techniques need to be studied with the involvement of the ethnic community members in general and specific variations within the subgroups identified for tailor-made intervention techniques. The service user, family members and carers also need to become integral parts of the health service management in mental health settings, including care plans. This has been observed to be highly inadequate in practice in England, as it has been found that more than one quarter of care plans did not include inputs from the patients (Care Quality Commission, CQC, 2013).

- The role of acculturation to mainstream society by migrant populations and indeed indigenous peoples), must also not be discounted in developed countries. Individuals who already experience perceived racism and challenge with 'fitting in' under 'normal' circumstances are likely to be more disempowered when they experience mental health challenges. Indeed, racism and racial discrimination have been credited with contributing to mental health problems; it, therefore, indicates that professionals need to consider this aspect as part of a holistic approach to their assessments, intervention, and care.
- It is, therefore, necessary for the current highly medical model prone system of care in mental health services to be completely overhauled in favour of a psycho-socio-cultural approach that takes into cognisance the influence of collective cultures in the individual's experience of care, control, and intricacies of power in mental health services, with a view to managing the intricacies to achieve good mental health outcomes. Mental health services also need to be taken into and embedded within the racialized communities, with

partnership with the voluntary sector organisations who have the knowledge and intelligence of the role and management of the historical-socio-cultural influences on wellbeing. This is the only way that the current state of poor experiences and poor statistics of mental health service users from ethnic communities with the Mental Health Services, the poor recovery levels and the overall over representation of this group in mental health settings could be stemmed.

2.4. Addendum - 2021 And Beyond

This chapter has been added before going to press in 2021.

The contents of the preceding chapters become quite poignant in view of the health and societal issues that have been unravelling before everyone's eyes since the outbreak of Covid-19 pandemic in 2020.

The indicators from more recent literature that buttresses findings and recommendations in preceding section/s include:

- The outbreak of Covid-19 in 2020 has disproportionately impacted on BAME communities in comparison to their White counterparts, in addition to the already prevailing experience higher levels of negative mental health outcomes for BAME groups in comparison to the general population in the United Kingdom, thereby worsening the inequalities (Smith et al, 2020; Iqbal, 2021; Proto & Quintana-Domeque, 2020)
- It has been more recently identified that internalised locus of control, financial challenges, and mental health intersects (Frankham et al, 2020). This accentuates the need for programmes that focuses on tackling inequality in access to employment for BME peoples to be a top priority as indicated in the previous chapters.
- As it has also been established that the quality of healthcare is 'significantly predicted' by "patients' ethnicity, language and culture" (Chauhan et al, 2020: 119).

Indeed, there has been no event in recent times that one could describe as unprecedented, considering the loss of lives from the virus outbreak in a worldwide context. The stark realities of the outbreak have not only demonstrated the vulnerabilities of all categories of the society at large but continue to echo the inequality in health outcomes in general and mental health for the BAME and CALD communities all over the world.

References

1. Abella, R. and Heslin, R. (1984) 'Health, Locus of Control, Values, and the Behavior of Family and Friends: An Integrated Approach to Understanding Preventive Health Behavior'. *Basic and Applied Social Psychology* 5 (4), 283-293
2. Adams, G. (2005) 'The Cultural Grounding of Personal Relationship: Enemyship in North American and West African Worlds'. *Journal of Personality and Social Psychology* 88, 948–968
3. Adebowale, L. (2013) *Independent Commission on Mental Health & Policing Report.* Available from: news.bbc.co.uk/2/shared/bsp/hi/pdfs/10_05_13_report.pdf
4. Aguiar de Sousa, L. (2017) *Merleau-Ponty on Temporality and Subjectivity in the Phenomenology of Perception* [online] available from <https://www.academia.edu/32298016/Merleau-Ponty_on_Temporality_and_Subjectivity_in_the_Phenomenology_of_Perception
5. Agyemang, C., Bhopal, R., and Bruijnzeels, M. (2005) 'Negro, Black, Black African, African Caribbean, African American or what? Labelling African Origin Populations in the Health Arena in the 21st Century' *J Epidemiol Community Health* 59, 1014–1018
6. Akande, A. and Lester, D. (1994) 'Suicidal Preoccupation, Depression and Locus of Control in Nigerians and Americans'. *Personality and Individual Differences* 16 (6), 979-988
7. Allan, H. T, and Westwood, S. (2015) 'White British researchers and internationally educated research participants: Insights from reflective practices on issues of language and culture in nursing contexts' *Journal of Research in Nursing* 20 (8), 640–652
8. Allen, D. E., de Nesnera, A., and Souther, J. W. (2009) 'Executive-Level Reviews of Seclusion and Restraint Promote

Interdisciplinary Collaboration and Innovation'. *Journal of the American Psychiatric Nurses Association* 15 (4), 260-264

9. Alshenqeeti, H. (2014) 'Interviewing as a Data Collection Method: A Critical Review'. *English Linguistics Research* 3 (1), 39-45
10. Anderson, L. (2008) Reflexivity. In: Thorpe R, Holt R, eds. *The Sage Dictionary of Qualitative Management Research*. Sage, London: 183–185
11. Arain, M., Campbell, M. J., Cooper, C. L., and Lancaster, G. A. (2010) 'What is a Pilot Or Feasibility Study? A Review of Current Practice and Editorial Policy'. *BMC Medical Research Methodology* 10 (67), 1-7
12. Arnold, E. (2012) *Working with Families of African Caribbean Origin – Understanding the Issues around Immigration and Attachment.* UK: Jessica Kingsley Publishers
13. Avtgis, T. A., Brann, M., and Staggers, S. M. (2006) 'Perceived Information Exchange and Health Control Expectancies as Influenced by a Patient's Medical Interview Situation'. *Communication Research Reports* 23 (4), 231-237
14. Avtgis, T. A. (1998) 'Locus of Control and Persuasion, Social Influence, and Conformity: A Meta-Analytic Review'. *Psychological Reports* 83 (3), 899-903
15. Bailis, D. S., Segall, A., and Chipperfield, J. G. (2010) 'Age, Relative Autonomy and Change in Health Locus of Control Beliefs: A Longitudinal Study of Members of a Health-Promotion Facility'. *Journal of Health Psychology* 15 (3), 326-338
16. Bains, J. (2005) 'Race, Culture and Psychiatry: A History of Transcultural Psychiatry'. *History of Psychiatry* 16 (2), 139-154
17. Ballard, R. (2002) 'Race, Ethnicity and Culture'. In *New Directions in Sociology*. ed. by Holborn, M. Ormskirk: Causeway.
18. Bandura, A. (1977) *Social Learning Theory*. Englewood Cliffs, NJ: Prentice Hall.
19. Baranowski, T. (1984) 'Social Support and Health Related Behavior Change Maintenance'. *Society for the Advancement of Social Psychology Newsletter* 10 (1), 13-15

20. Barber, P. Brown, R., & Martin, D. (2012) *Mental Health Law in England and Wales: A Guide to Mental Health Professionals.* 2nd edn. London: Sage
21. Barkhan, S. E. (2012) 'Theories of Power and Society'. In *Sociology: Comprehensive Edition (V. 1.0).* Available from: https://2012books.lardbucket.org/books/sociology-comprehensive-edition/s17-03-theories-of-power-and-society.html
22. Barroso, J., McMillan, S., Casey, L., Gibson, W., Kaminski, G., and Meyer, J. (2000) 'Comparison between African-American and White Women in their Beliefs about Breast Cancer and their Health Locus of Control'. *Cancer Nursing* 23 (4), 268-276
23. Barry, J. (2013) *Theories of Power: Pluralist, Elitist and Marxist Perspectives* available from <https://www.academia.edu/3270103/Theories_of_Power_Pluralist_Elitist_and_Marxist_Perspectives?Auto=download> []
24. Benassi, V. A., Sweeney, P. D., and Dufour, C. L. (1988) 'Is there a Relation between Locus of Control Orientation and Depression?'. *Journal of Abnormal Psychology* 97 (3), 357-367
25. Bennett, J. and Keating, F. (2009) 'Training to Redress Racial Disadvantage in Mental Health Care: Race Equality Or Cultural Competence?' *Journal of Public Mental Health* 8 (2), 40–46
26. Bennett, M. (1993) 'Towards Ethnorelativism: A Developmental Model of Intercultural Sensitivity'. in *Education for the Intercultural Experience*. ed. by Paige, R. M. Yarmouth, Me: Intercultural Press, 21-71
27. Bennett, P., Norman, P., Moore, L., Murphy, S., and Tudor-Smith, C. (1997) 'Health Locus of Control and Value for Health in Smokers and Nonsmokers'. *Health Psychology: Official Journal of the Division of Health Psychology, American Psychological Association* 16 (2), 179-182
28. Bergin, M., Wells, J. S. G., and Owen, S. (2008) 'Critical Realism: A Philosophical Framework for the Study of Gender and Mental Health'. *Nursing Philosophy: An International Journal for Healthcare Professionals* 9 (3), 169-179

29. Bernard, C. and Gupta, A. (2008) 'Black African Children and the Child Protection System'. *The British Journal of Social Work* 38 (3), 476-492
30. Bernard, H. R. (2002) *Research Methods in Anthropology: Qualitative and Quantitative Approaches*. 3rd edn. Walnut Creek, CA: Alta Mira Press
31. Bhaskar, R. and Danermark, B. (2006) 'Metatheory, Interdisciplinarity and Disability Research: A Critical Realist Perspective'. *Scandinavian Journal of Disability Research* 8 (4), 278-297
32. Bhaumik, S. (2012) 'Negotiating Diversity in Clinical Care: A Guide for Service Organisations and Clinicians' Available from: www.rcpsych.ac.uk/pdf/15%20Bhaumik%20IC2012.pdf
33. Bhopal, K. (2010) 'Gender, identity and experience: Researching marginalised groups' *Women's Studies International Forum* 33 (3), 188-195
34. Bhopal, R. (2004) 'Glossary of Terms Relating to Ethnicity and Race: For Reflection and Debate'. *Journal of Epidemiology and Community Health* 58 (6), 441-445
35. Bhugra, D, Bahl, V. (1999) *Ethnicity: An Agenda for Mental Health. Gaskell, London Royal College of Psychiatrists:* Gaskell, London Royal College of Psychiatrists.
36. Bhui, K., Brown, P., Hardie, T., Watson, J. P., and Parrott, J. (1998) 'African-Caribbean Men Remanded to Brixton Prison. Psychiatric and Forensic Characteristics and Outcome of Final Court Appearance'. *The British Journal of Psychiatry: The Journal of Mental Science* 172, 337-344
37. Bhui, K, Bhugra, D. (2002) 'Mental Illness in Black and Asian Ethnic Minority: Pathways to Care and Outcomes'. *Advances in Psychiatric Treatment* 8, 26-33
38. Bhui, K., O'Hara, J. (2014) 'Ethnic Inequalities, Complexity and Social Exclusion'. In *Annual Report of the Chief Medical Officer 2013. Public Mental Health Priorities: Investing in Evidence*. ed. by Davies, S. C. London: Department of Health, 276–284

39. Bhui, K., Ullrich, S., and Coid, J. W. (2014) 'Which Pathways to Psychiatric Care Lead to Earlier Treatment and a Shorter Duration of First-Episode Psychosis?' *BMC Psychiatry* 14 (72), 1-11
40. Bhui, K., McCabe, R., Weich, S., Singh, S., Johnson, M., and Szczepura, A. (2013) 'THERACOM: A Systematic Review of the Evidence Base for Interventions to Improve Therapeutic Communications between Black and Minority Ethnic Populations and Staff in Specialist Mental Health Services'. *Systematic Reviews* 2 (15), 1-11
41. Bhui, K., Stansfeld, S., Hull, S., Priebe, S., Mole, F., and Feder, G. (2003) 'Ethnic Variations in Pathways to and use of Specialist Mental Health Services in the UK: Systematic Review'. *The British Journal of Psychiatry* 182 (2), 105-116
42. Bhui, K. S. and Singh, S. P. (2004) 'Introduction: Cultural Psychiatry Research for the Next Decade'. *Journal of Mental Health* 13 (2), 125-127
43. Bishop, F., and Holmes, M. (2013) ‘Mixed Methods in CAM Research: A Systematic Review of Studies’ *Evid Based Complement Alternat Med* Available from <http://dx.doi.org/10.1155/2013/187365>
44. Bonsack, C. and Borgeat, F. (2005) 'Perceived Coercion and Need for Hospitalization Related to Psychiatric Admission'. *International Journal of Law and Psychiatry* 28 (4), 342-347
45. Borrell-Carrió, F., Suchman, A. L., and Epstein, R. M. (2004) 'The Biopsychosocial Model 25 Years Later: Principles, Practice, and Scientific Inquiry'. *The Annals of Family Medicine* 2 (6), 576-582
46. Bradby, H. (2010) 'Institutional Racism in Mental Health Services: The Consequences of Compromised Conceptualisation'. *Sociological Research Online* 15 (3), 1-11
47. Bradley, K. (2009) *The Bradley Report: Lord Bradley’s Review of Groups with Mental Health Problems Or Learning Disabilities in the Criminal Justice System* Available from: www.centreformentalhealth.org.uk/pdfs/Bradley_report_2009.pdf

48. Brilowski, G.A., & Wendler M.C. (2005) 'An Evolutionary Concept Analysis of Caring'. *Journal of Advanced Nursing* 50 (6), 641-650
49. British Sociological Association (2017) *Language and the BSA: Ethnicity & Race* [online] available from <https://nanopdf.com/download/language-and-the-bsa-ethnicity-amp-race_pdf>
50. Brocki, J. M. and Wearden, A. J. (2006) 'A Critical Evaluation of the use of Interpretative Phenomenological Analysis (IPA) in Health Psychology'. *Psychology & Health* 21 (1), 87-108
51. Broer, T., Nieboer, A. P., and Bal, R. (2012) 'Governing Mental Health Care: How Power is Exerted in and through a Quality Improvement Collaborative'. *Public Administration* 90 (3), 800-815
52. Broom, A. and Willis, E. (2007) *Competing Paradigms and Health Research* in Researching Health. Qualitative, Quantitative and Mixed Methods. ed. by Saks, M, Allsop, J., Thousand Oaks, CA: Sage, 16–31
53. Brough, J.B, Blattner, W. (2006) 'Temporality'. In *A Companion to Phenomenology and Existentialism*. ed. by Dreyfus, H.L, Wrathall, M.A.: Blackwell Publishing
54. Brown, D. and Edwards, H. E. (2008) *Lewis's Medical-Surgical Nursing: Assessment and Management of Clinical Problems [2nd Ed.]*. Marrickville, N.S.W: Elsevier.
55. Brown, N., Muhlenkamp, A., Fox, L., and Osborn, M. (1983) 'The Relationship among Health Beliefs, Health Values, and Health Promotion Activity'. *Western Journal of Nursing Research* 5 (2), 155-163
56. Brown, R. (2016) *The Approved Mental Health Professional's Guide to Mental Health Law*. 4th edn. UK: SAGE
57. Brown, S. (2016) 'Mental Capacity and Social Policy'. In *Policy and Social Work Practice*. ed. by Evans, T, Keating F. London: SAGE Publications Ltd, 99
58. Buhagiar, K., Parsonage, L., and Osborn, D. P. J. (2011) 'Physical Health Behaviours and Health Locus of Control in People with Schizophrenia-Spectrum Disorder and Bipolar Disorder: A Cross-

Sectional Comparative Study with People with Non-Psychotic Mental Illness'. *BMC Psychiatry* 11 (104), 1-10

59. Burgoyne, R. W., Staples, F. R., Yamamoto, J., Wolkon, G. H., and Kline, F. (1979) 'Patients' Requests of an Outpatient Clinic'. *Archives of General Psychiatry* 36 (4), 400-403
60. Burk, C, and Kimiecik, J. (1994) 'Examining the Relationship among Locus of Control, Health Value and Exercise'. *Health Values* 18, 14-23
61. Campbell, C., Cornish, F., and Mclean, C. (2004) 'Social Capital, Participation and the Perpetuation of Health Inequalities: Obstacles to African-Caribbean Participation in 'Partnerships' to Improve Mental Health'. *Ethnicity & Health* 9 (4), 313-335
62. Cantor-Graae, E. (2007) 'Ethnic Minority Groups, Particularly African-Caribbean and Black African Groups, are at Increased Risk of Psychosis in the UK'. *Evidence-Based Mental Health* 10 (3), 95
63. Cappuccio, F.P., Cooj, D. G., Atkinson, R.W., et al. (1998) 'The Wandsworth Heart and Stroke Study. A Population-Based Survey of Cardiovascular Risk Factors in Different Ethnic Groups. Methods and Baseline Findings'. *Nutr Metab Cardiovasc Dis* 8, 371–385
64. Care Quality Commission (2017) *The State of Care in Mental Health Services 2014 to 2017*: Care Quality Commission. Available from: http://www.cqc.org.uk/sites/default/files/20170720_stateofmh_report.pdf
65. Care Quality Commission (2016) *Monitoring the Mental Health Act in 2015/16*: Care Quality Commission. Available from: http://www.cqc.org.uk/sites/default/files/20161122_mhareport1516_web.pdf
66. Care Quality Commission (2014) *Monitoring the Mental Health Act in 2012/13.* : Care Quality Commission. Available from: http://www.cqc.org.uk/sites/default/files/documents/cqc_mentalhealth_2012_13_07_update.pdf

67. Care Quality Commission (2011) *Count Me in 2010: Results of the 2010 National Census of Inpatients and Patients on Supervised Community Treatment in Mental Health and Learning Disability Services in England and Wales*: Care Quality Commission. Available from: www.cqc.org.uk/sites/default/files/.../count_me_in_2010_final_tagged.pdf
68. Carling, J., Erdal, M. B., and Ezzati, R. (2013) 'Beyond the insider–outsider divide in migration research' *Migration Studies* 2 (1), 36–54
69. Carpenter, S. (2000) 'Effects of Cultural Tightness and Collectivism on Self-Concept and Causal Attributions'. *Cross-Cultural Research* 34 (1), 38-56
70. Centre for Mental Health (2017) *Against the Odds: Evaluation of the Mind Birmingham Up My Street Programme.* Available from *<https://www.centreformentalhealth.org.uk/Handlers/Download.ashx?IDMF=14f86686-7882-43cb-b64e-1540f12ab01a>*
71. Chapman, M., Skinner, E. A., Bakes, P. B. (1990) 'Interpreting Correlations between Children's Perceived Control and Cognitive Performance: Control, Agency, Or Means-Ends Beliefs?'. *Developmental Psychology* 26 (2), 246-253
72. Charmaz, K. (2000). Grounded theory. In N.K. Denzin, & Y.S. Lincoln (Eds.), 'Handbook of Qualitative Research' (2nd ed) Thousand Oaks, Ca: Sage
73. Chaturvedi, N., McKeigue, P. M., and Marmot, M. G. (1993) 'Resting and Ambulatory Blood Pressure Differences in Afro-Caribbeans and Europeans'. *Hypertension (Dallas, Tex.: 1979)* 22 (1), 90-96
74. Chauhan, A., Walton, M., Manias, E. et al(2020). The safety of health care for ethnic minority patients: a systematic review. Int J Equity Health 19, 118
75. Chen, S., Acton, G., and Shao, J. (2010) 'Relationships among Nutritional Self-Efficacy, Health Locus of Control and Nutritional Status in Older Taiwanese Adults'. *Journal of Clinical Nursing* 19 (15-16), 2117-2127

76. Cheng, C., Cheung, S., Chio, J. H., and Chan, M. S. (2013) 'Cultural Meaning of Perceived Control: A Meta-Analysis of Locus of Control and Psychological Symptoms Across 18 Cultural Regions'. *Psychological Bulletin* 139 (1), 152-188
77. Clarke, C. (2009) 'An Introduction to Interpretative Phenomenological Analysis: A Useful Approach for Occupational Therapy Research'. *The British Journal of Occupational Therapy* 72 (1), 37-39
78. Cohen, M. A. and Dennett, D. C. (2011) 'Consciousness Cannot be Separated from Function'. *Trends in Cognitive Sciences* 15 (8), 358-364
79. Commission for Healthcare Audit and Inspection (2007) *Count Me in: Results of the 2006 National Census of Inpatients in Mental Health and Learning Disability Services in England and Wales.* London: Commission for Healthcare Audit and Inspection
80. Cornish, F. and Gillespie, A. (2009) 'A Pragmatist Approach to the Problem of Knowledge in Health Psychology'. *Journal of Health Psychology* 14 (6), 800-809
81. Craig, G., Atkin, K., Chattoo, S., and Flynn, R. (2012) *Understanding 'Race' and Ethnicity: Theory, History, Policy, Practice* 1st edn. University of Bristol: Policy Press
82. Cresswell, J. W., & Plano, C. V. L. (2011) *Designing and Conducting Mixed Methods Research* 2nd edn. CA: Thousand Oaks. Sage
83. Creswell, J. W. (2009) *Research Design: Qualitative, Quantitative and Mixed Methods Approach* 3rd edn. UK: SAGE.
84. Crisp, N., Smith, G. and Nicholson, K. (2016) *Old Problems, New Solutions: Improving Acute Psychiatric Care for Adults in England:* The Commission on Acute Adult Psychiatric Care] available from <http://media.wix.com/ugd/0e662e_aaca63ae4737410e9e2873 dfde849841.pdf
85. Cruickshank, J. K., Cooper, J., Burnett, M., MacDuff, J., and Drubra, U. (1991) 'Ethnic Differences in Fasting Plasma C-Peptide and Insulin in Relation to Glucose Tolerance and Blood Pressure'. *Lancet,* 338 (8771), 842-847

86. Culley L, Hudson, N., and Rapport F. (2007) 'Using focus groups with minority ethnic communities: Researching infertility in British South Asian communities' *Qualitative Health Research* 17 (1), 102–112
87. Darawsheh, W (2014) 'Reflexivity in research: Promoting rigour, reliability and validity in qualitative research' *International Journal of Therapy and Rehabilitation* 21 (12), 560-568
88. Davies, S., Thornicroft, G., Leese, M., Higgingbotham, A., and Phelan, M. (1996) 'Ethnic Differences in Risk of Compulsory Psychiatric Admission among Representative Cases of Psychosis in London'. *BMJ (Clinical Research Ed.)* 312 (7030), 533-537
89. Declerck, C., De Brabander, B., Boone, C., and Gerits, P. (2002) 'Locus of Control, Marital Status and Predictors of Early Relapse in Primary Breast Cancer Patients'. *Psychology & Health* 17 (1), 63-76
90. Declerck, C. H., Boone, C., and De Brabander, B. (2006) 'On Feeling in Control: A Biological Theory for Individual Differences in Control Perception'. *Brain and Cognition* 62 (2), 143-176
91. Dein, S. and Bhui, K. S. (2013) 'At the Crossroads of Anthropology and Epidemiology: Current Research in Cultural Psychiatry in the UK'. *Transcultural Psychiatry* 50 (6), 769-791
92. Dennis, S. (1997) 'Close Observation: How to Improve Assessments'. *Nursing Times* 93 (24), 54-56
93. Denzin, N.K., Lincoln, Y. S (2005) *The Sage Handbook of Qualitative Research* (3rd edition) Thousand Oaks, Sage
94. Department of Health (2017a) *Terms of Reference – Independent Review of the Mental Health Act 1983.* Department of Health
95. Department of Health (2017b) *The Government's Response to the Five Year Forward View for Mental Health:* Department of Health. Available from <https://www.gov.uk/government/uploads/system/uploads/attachment_data/file/582120/FYFV_mental_health__government_response.pdf>
96. Department of Health (2015) *Code of Practice Mental Health Act 1983*. London: Department of Health Department of Health

(2014a) *Achieving Better Access to Mental Health Services by 2020.* Available from <https://www.gov.uk/government/uploads/system/uploads/attachment_data/file/361648/mental-health-access.pdf>

97. Department of Health (2014b) *The Care Act. 2014*: Department of Health
98. Department of Health (2014c) *Closing the gap: priorities for essential change in mental health*. Available from <https://www.gov.uk/government/uploads/system/uploads/attachment_data/file/281250/Closing_the_gap_V2_-_17_Feb_2014.pdf
99. Department of Health (2013) *Annual Report of the Chief Medical Officer 2013, Public Mental Health Priorities: Investing in the Evidence.:* Department of Health Available from <https://www.gov.uk/government/uploads/system/uploads/attachment_data/file/413196/CMO_web_doc.pdf>
100. Department of Health (2011) *No Health without Mental Health. Delivering Better Mental Health Outcomes for Groups of all Ages. London:* Department of Health. Available from <National archives: www.nationalarchives.gov.uk/doc/open-government-licence/>
101. Department of Health (2010) *National Mental Health and Learning Disability Ethnicity Census: Count Me in 2010.* London: Care Quality Commission (CQC) & National Mental Health Development Unit (NMHDU).
102. Department of Health (2005a) *Delivering Race Equality in Mental Health Care – an Action Plan for Reform Inside and Outside Services and Independent Inquiry into the Death of David Bennett in Mental Health Care.* Available from <http://webarchive.nationalarchives.gov.uk/20130107105354/http:/www.dh.gov.uk/en/publicationsandstatistics/publications/publicationspolicyandguidance/dh_4100773>
103. Department of Health (2005b) *Delivering Race Equality in Mental Health Care: An Action Plan for Reform Inside and Outside Services and the Government's Response to the*

Independent Inquiry into the Death of David Bennett. London: Department of Health. Available from<http://www.dh.gov.uk/en/Publicationsandstatistics/Publications/PublicationsPolicyandGuidance/DH_4100773>

104. Department of Health (2003) *Delivering Race Equality: A Framework for Action, Mental Health Services Consultation Document*. London: Department of Health
105. Diclemente, C. C. (1986) 'Self-Efficacy and the Addictive Behaviors'. *Journal of Social and Clinical Psychology* 4 (3), 302-315
106. Dijkstraa M. T. M, Beersma, B, and Evers, A (2011) 'Reducing Conflict-Related Employee Strain: The Benefits of an Internal Locus of Control and a Problem Solving Conflict Management Strategy'. *Work and Stress* 25, 167- 84
107. Donovan, D. M. and O'Leary, M. R. (1978) 'The Drinking-Related Locus of Control Scale. Reliability, Factor Structure and Validity'. *Journal of Studies on Alcohol* 39 (5), 759-784
108. Duffy, D. (1995) 'Out of the Shadows: A Study of the Special Observation of Suicidal Psychiatric In-Patients'. *Journal of Advanced Nursing* 21 (5), 944-950
109. Duffy, M. E. (1988) 'Determinants of Health Promotion in Midlife Women'. *Nursing Research* 37 (6), 358-362
110. Edge, D. and West, W. (2011) 'Mental Health and 'The Big Society': Where do Counselling Psychologists and Therapists Fit in?'. *Counselling Psychology Review* 26 (2), 17-23
111. Edge, D., Degnan, A., Cotterill, S., Berry, K., Drake, R., Baker, J., Barrowclough, C., Hughes-Morley, A., Grey, P., Bhugra, D., Cahoon, P., Tarrier, N., Lewis, S., and Abel, K. (2016) 'Culturally-Adapted Family Intervention (CaFI) for African-Caribbeans Diagnosed with Schizophrenia and their Families: A Feasibility Study Protocol of Implementation and Acceptability'. *Pilot and Feasibility Studies* 2 (39), 1-14
112. Edge, D. (2013) 'Why are You Cast Down, O My Soul? Exploring Intersections of Ethnicity, Gender, Depression, Spirituality and

Implications for Black British Caribbean Women's Mental Health'. *Critical Public Health* 23 (1), 39-48

113. Edge, D. (2011) "It's Leaflet, Leaflet, Leaflet then, "See You Later"': Black Caribbean Women's Perceptions of Perinatal Mental Health Care'. *The British Journal of General Practice: The Journal of the Royal College of General Practitioners* 61 (585), 256-262
114. Edge, D. (2010) 'Falling through the Net - Black and Minority Ethnic Women and Perinatal Mental Healthcare: Health Professionals' Views'. *General Hospital Psychiatry* 32 (1), 17-25
115. Edge, D. and MacKian, S. C. (2010) 'Ethnicity and Mental Health Encounters in Primary Care: Help-Seeking and Help-Giving for Perinatal Depression among Black Caribbean Women in the UK'. *Ethnicity & Health* 15 (1), 93-111
116. Edge, D. (2008) "We Don't See Black Women here': An Exploration of the Absence of Black Caribbean Women from Clinical and Epidemiological Data on Perinatal Depression in the UK'. *Midwifery* 24 (4), 379-389
117. Edge, D. (2007) 'Ethnicity, Psychosocial Risk, and Perinatal Depression--a Comparative Study among Inner-City Women in the United Kingdom'. *Journal of Psychosomatic Research* 63 (3), 291-295
118. Edge, D. and Rogers, A. (2005) 'Dealing with it: Black Caribbean Women's Response to Adversity and Psychological Distress Associated with Pregnancy, Childbirth, and Early Motherhood'. *Social Science & Medicine* 61 (1), 15-25
119. Egharevba I. (2001) 'Researching an-'other' minority ethnic community: Reflections of a black female researcher on the intersections of race, gender and other power positions on the research process' *International Journal of Social Research Methodology*, 4 (3), 225-241
120. Elder, R., Evans, K., Nizette, D. (2009) *Psychiatric and Mental Health Nursing.* 2nd edn. Australia.: Elsevier
121. Elliott, J. G. C. (1993) *Locus of Control in Children with Emotional and Behavioural*

Difficulties: An Exploratory Study.; [online] thesis or dissertation. Available from Durham E-Theses Online: http://etheses.dur.ac.uk/1619/

122. Engel, G. L. (2004) 'The need for a new medical model: A challenge for Biomedicine', in Health, Disease and Illness, Concepts in Medicine. Ed. By Caplan, A.L., McCartney, J.J., Sisti, D. A. U.S.A: Georgetown University Press. 7, 51-64.
123. Evans, A., Hardy, M., and Shaw, I. (2010) *Evidence and Knowledge for Practice.* Cambridge: Polity Press
124. Evans, T, Keating, F (2016) *Policy and Social Work Practice* London: SAGE.
125. Fade, S. (2004) 'Using Interpretative Phenomenological Analysis for Public Health Nutrition and Dietetic Research: A Practical Guide'. *The Proceedings of the Nutrition Society* 63 (4), 647-653
126. Fearon, P., Kirkbride, J. B., Morgan, C., Dazzan, P., Morgan, K., Lloyd, T., Hutchinson, G., Tarrant, J., Fung, W. L. A., Holloway, J., Mallett, R., Harrison, G., Leff, J., Jones, P. B., and Murray, R. M. (2006) 'Incidence of Schizophrenia and Other Psychoses in Ethnic Minority Groups: Results from the MRC AESOP Study'. *Psychological Medicine* 36 (11), 1541-1550
127. Fernando, S. (1998) 'Studies into Issues of 'Race' and Culture in Psychiatry'. *Psychological Medicine* 28 (2), 496-497
128. Fernando, S. (1995) *Mental Health in a Multi-Ethnic Society: A Multi-Disciplinary Handbook.* London: Routledge.
129. Fernando, S. (1991) *Mental Health, Race and Culture.* Basingstoke: Macmillan / Mind
130. Fernando, S., Keating, F. (2009) *Mental Health in a Multi-Ethnic Society: A Multidisciplinary Handbook.* Hove: Routledge
131. Flanagan, S. M., and Hancock, B (2010) ''Reaching the hard to reach' - lessons learned from the
132. VCS (voluntary and community Sector). A qualitative study' *BMC Health Serv Res.* 10 (92), 1-9
133. Foucault, M. (2010) *The Government of Self and Others. Lectures at the College De France, 1982–1983.* Basingstoke: Palgrave Macmillan.

134. Foucault, M. (2006) *History of Madness.* London and New York: Routledge.
135. Foucault, M. (2001) *Madness and Civilisation: A History of Insanity in the Age of Reason.:* London: Routledge Classic
136. Foucault, M. (1986) *The Care of the Self, the History of Sexuality 3.* New York: Vintage Books
137. Foucault, M. (1985) *The use of Pleasure, the History of Sexuality 2.* New York: Vintage Books.
138. Foucault, M. (1980) 'The Eye of Power'. in *Power/Knowledge.* ed. by Gordon, C. Bnghton: Harvester
139. Foucault, M. (1977) *Discipline and Punish: The Birth of the Prison.* London: Penguin Books
140. Fox, N. (1995) 'Postmodern Perspectives on Care: The Vigil and the Gift'. *Critical Social Policy* 4/5 (15), 125.
141. Frankham, C., Richardson, T. & Maguire, N (2020). Do Locus of Control, Self-esteem, Hope and
142. Shame Mediate the Relationship Between Financial Hardship and Mental Health?. *Community Ment Health,* **56,** 404–415.
143. Fuchs, T., Van Duppen, Z. (2017) Time and Events: On the Phenomenology of Temporal Experience in Schizophrenia (Ancillary Article to EAWE Domain 2).' *Psychopathology. Available at: https://www.academia.edu/2027576/The_three_levels_of_temporality_in_Husserlian_phenomenology*
144. Furnham, A. (1983) 'The A Type Behaviour Pattern, Mental Health and Health Locus of Control Beliefs'. *Social Science & Medicine* 17 (20), 1569–1572.
145. Furnham, A. C., E. (2004) 'Lay Theories of Schizophrenia: A Cross-Cultural Comparison of British and Hong Kong Chinese Attitudes, Attributions and Beliefs'. *Social Psychiatry and Psychiatric Epidemiology* (39), 543-552
146. Garcia-Toro, M., Aguirre, I. (2007) 'Biopsychosocial Model in Depression Revisited.'. *Medical Hypotheses* 68, 683–691
147. Gardner, K. (1992) 'The Historical Conflict between Caring and Professionalization, a Dilemma for Nursing'. In *The Presence of*

Caring. ed. by Gaut, D. A. New York: National League for Nursing Press.

148. Garland, J., Spalek, B., and Chakraborti, N (2006) 'Hearing Lost Voices: Issues in Researching 'Hidden' Minority Ethnic Communities' *The British Journal of Criminology*, 46 (3), 423–437Georgiou, A. and Bradley, C. (1992) 'The Development of a Smoking-Specific Locus of Control Scale'. *Psychology & Health* 6 (3), 227-240
149. Gillis A., J. W. (2002) 'Introduction to Nursing Research'. In *Research for Nurses: Method and Interpretation*. ed. by Gillis A. Jackson W. Philadelphia: F. A. Davis, 3-36
150. Glasser, I., Bridgeman, R. (1999) *Braving the Street: The Anthropology of Homelessness.* New York: Berghahn Books.
151. Golightley, M. (2014) *Social Work and Mental Health.* 5th edition. Exeter: Learning Matters
152. Graham, H. (1983) 'Caring: A Labour of Love'. In *A Labour of Love: Women, Work and Caring*. ed. by Finch, J, Groves, D. London: Routledge and Kegan Paul
153. Graham, H. (1991) 'The Concept of Caring in Feminist Research: The Case of Domestic Service'. *Sociology* 25 (1), 61-78
154. Graham, M. (2002) 'Creating Spaces: Exploring the Role of Cultural Knowledge as a Source of Empowerment in Models of Social Welfare in Black Communities'. *The British Journal of Social Work* 32 (1), 35-49
155. Green, J., and Thorogood, N. (2004) *Qualitative Methods for Health Research*. London: Sage Publications
156. Grigg, M. (2006) 'Eliminating Seclusion and Restraint in Australia'. *International Journal of Mental Health Nursing* 15, 224-225.
157. Gupta, A., Featherstone, B. (2015) 'What about My Dad? Black Fathers and the Child Protection System'. *Critical and Radical Social Work* 4 (1), 77-91
158. Haines, A. P., Booroff, A., Goldenberg, E., Morgan, P., Singh, M., and Wallace, P. (1987) 'Blood Pressure, Smoking, Obesity and

Alcohol Consumption in Black and White Patients in General Practice'. *Journal of Human Hypertension* 1 (1), 39-46

159. Hall, S. (1993) 'Culture, Community, Nation'. *Cultural Studies* 7 (3), 349-363
160. Halpert, R., and Hill, R. (2011) *28 Measures of Locus of Control.* Available at: http://teachinternalcontrol.com/uploads/LOC_Measures__1_.pdf
161. Hamilton, B. and Love, A. (2010) 'Reducing Reliance on Seclusion in Acute Psychiatry'. *Australian Nursing Journal* 18 (3), 43
162. Hamilton, J. P. (1991) 'The Development of a Communication Specific Locus of Control Instrument'. *Communication Reports* 4 (2), 108-112
163. Hampson, S.E. (1995) *The Construction of Personality* (2nd ed.) London: Routledge
164. Hardy, M. (2015) *Governing risk: care and control in contemporary social work*. UK: Palgrave Macmillan
165. Hardy, M. (2016) 'Discretion in the History and Development of Social Work'. In *Policy and Social Work Practice.* ed. by Evans, T, Keating, F, London: SAGE.
166. Haslam, S.A., Jetten, J., Postmes, T., and Haslam, C, (2009) 'Social Identity, Health and Well-Being: An Emerging Agenda for Applied Psychology'. *Applied Psychology: An International Review* 58 (1), 1–23
167. Hess, M, and Vossel, G. (2001) 'Stress, resources and coping behaviour in the assessment center-participants' reactions. *Zeitschrift fur Arbeitsund organisation psychologie* 45, 202–210
168. Hewitt, M. (2009) *Reviewing and Evaluating Literature. The NIHR Research Design Service for Yorkshire & the Humber, Resource Pack*. Available from: https://www.worcester.ac.uk/documents/6_Critically_evaluate_research_literature_2009v2.pdf

169. Hill, D.J. and Bale, R.M. (1980) 'Development of the Mental Health Locus of Control and Mental Health Locus of Origin Scales' *Journal of Personality Assessment* 44 (2), 148-156
170. Holder, E. E. and Levi, D. J. (1988) 'Mental health and locus of control: SCL-90-R and Levenson's IPC scales'. *Journal of Clinical Psychology* 44, 753–755
171. Hough, L. M. (1992) 'The "Big Five" personality variables—construct confusion: Description versus prediction'. *Human Performance* 5, 139-155
172. Høyer, G., Kjellin, L., Engberg, M., Kaltiala-Heinod, R., Nilstune, T., Sigurjonsdottir, M., and Syse, A. (2002) 'Paternalism and autonomy: A presentation of a Nordic study on the use of coercion in the mental health care system'. *International Journal of Law and Psychiatry* 25, 93–108
173. Hugman, R. (1991) *Power in Caring Professions.* London: The Macmillan Press Limited
174. Hui, A. and Stickley, T. (2007) 'Mental health policy and mental health service user perspectives on involvement: a discourse analysis'. *Journal of Advanced Nursing* 59 (4), 416–426
175. Huizink, A. C., de Medina, P. G. R., Mulder, E. J. H., Visser, G. H. A., and Buitelaar, J. K. (2002) 'Coping in normal pregnancy'. *Annals of Behavioral Medicine* 24, 132–140
176. Hutchison, D. (2007. *The role of self-efficacy, locus of control, and intellectual ability in guided self-help for depression, anxiety and stress*. [Online] thesis or dissertation. Available from: British Library Electronic Theses Online Service- EThOS
177. Iqbal, N.(2021). Minority Mental Health: Intersections between Faith and Ethnicity Available at:
SSRN: https://ssrn.com/abstract=3767398 or http://dx.doi.org/10.2139/ssrn.3767398
178. Independent Police Complaints Commission (2011) *Deaths in custody study.* Available from: http://www.ipcc.gov.uk/page/deaths-custody-study

179. Iversen, K., Høyer, G., Sexton, H., and Grønli, O. K. (2002) 'Perceived Coercion among Patients Admitted to Acute Wards in Norway'. *Nordic Journal of Psychiatry* 56 (6), 433-439
180. Iversen, K. I., Høyer, G., and Sexton, H. C. (2007) 'Coercion and Patient Satisfaction on Psychiatric Acute Wards'. *International Journal of Law and Psychiatry* 30 (6), 504-511
181. Jones, R. (2011) *Mental Health Act Manual*. 14th edn. London: Sweet & Maxwell
182. Judge, T. A., Erez, A., Bono, J. E., and Thoresen, C. J. (2002) 'Are Measures of Self-Esteem, Neuroticism, Locus of Control, and Generalized Self-Efficacy Indicators of a Common Core Construct?'. *Journal of Personality and Social Psychology* 83 (3), 693-710
183. Joseph, S. (2018). Exploring the relationship between Locus of Control and the perception of the quality of mental health care experienced by African & Caribbean service users. Thesis or dissertation. Available at: pure.royalholloway.ac.uk
184. Jupp, V. (2005) 'Issues of Power in Social Work Practice in Mental Health Services for People from Black and Minority Ethnic Groups'. *Critical Social Work* 6. Available at: http://www1.uwindsor.ca/criticalsocialwork/issues-of-power-in-social-work-practice-in-mental-health-services-for-groups-from-black-and-minority
185. KalathiL, J. (2011) *Recovery and Resilience: African, African-Caribbean and Asian Women's Narratives of Recovering from Mental Distress*. London: Mental Health Foundation
186. Karlsen, S., Primatesta, P., McMum, A. (2001) 'Blood Pressure'. In *Health Survey for England—the Health of Minority Ethnic Groups '99*. ed. by Erens B, Primatesta P, Prior G. London: Stationery Office, 175–97
187. Keating, F. (2016) 'Racialised Communities, Producing Madness and Dangerousness'. *Intersectionalities: A Global Journal of Social Work Analysis, Research, Polity, and Practice* 5 (3), 1-13

188. Keating, F. (2016) 'Social Welfare Policy in Racialised Contexts'. In *Policy and Social Work Practice*. ed. by Evans, T, Keating, F. London: SAGE
189. Keating, F. (2012) 'Theorising 'Race', Ethnicity and Mental Health'. In *UNDERSTANDING 'RACE' AND ETHNICITY: Theory, History, Policy Practice*. ed. by Craig, G., Atkin, K., Chattoo, S. Flynn, R. Bristol: Policy Press, 209- 225
190. Keating, F, Robertson, D., McCulloch, A., Francis, E. (2002) *Breaking the Circles of Fear: A Review of the Relationship between Mental Health Services and African and Caribbean Communities*. London: The Sainsbury Centre for Mental Health
191. Keating, F. (2005) 'Social Inequalities and Mental Health: An Integrative Approach'. in *Beyond the Water Towers: The Unfinished Revolution in Mental Health Services 1985-2005*. ed. by Bell, A. London: Sainsbury Centre for Mental Health
192. Keating, F. and Robertson, D. (2004) 'Fear, Black People and Mental Illness: A Vicious
193. Circle?'. *Health & Social Care in the Community* 12 (5), 439-447
194. Kelley, J. A., St. Lawrence, J. S., Brasfield, T. L., Lemke, A., Amidei, T., Roffman, R. E., Hood, H.
195. V., Smith, J. E., Kilgore, H., and McNeill, C. (1990) 'Psychological factors that predict AIDS high-nsk versus AIDS precautionary behavior'. *Journal of Consulting and Clinical Psychology* 58, 117-120
196. Kesavayuth, D., Poyago-Theotoky, J., &Zikos, V. (2020), Locus of control, health and healthcare utilization. *Econ. Model.* 86, 227–238
197. Kirkcaldy, B. D., Shephard, R. J., and Funham, A. F. (2002) 'The influence of Type A behaviour and locus of control upon job satisfaction and occupational health'. *Personality and Individual Differences 33*, 1361–1371
198. Kirscht, J. P. (1972) 'Perceptions of control and health beliefs'. *Can. Journal of behav.* Sci./Rev. Canad. Sci. Comp 4 (3), 225-237
199. Kitzinger, J. (1995) 'Qualitative Research - Introducing Focus Groups' *British Medical Journal*

200. 311, 299-302

201. Knappe, S. and Pinquart, M. (2009) 'Tracing criteria of successful aging? Health Locus of Control and well-being in older patients with internal diseases'. *Psychology Health and Medicine* 14, 201-212

202. Kormanik, M. B, and Rocco, T. S. (2009) 'Internal versus external control of reinforcement: A review of the locus of control construct'. *Human Resource Development Review* 8, 463– 483

203. Kotecha N. (2008) 'Black and minority ethnic women'. In *Mental health in a multi-ethnic society: a multidisciplinary handbook.* ed. by Fernando S, Keating F. London: Routledge

204. Krueger, R, and Casey, M. (2000) *Focus Groups: A Practical Guide for Applied Research* (3rd ed.). Newbury Park, CA: Sage

205. Knight, M.T.D., Wykes, T., and Hayward, P. (2003) 'Groups don't understand': an investigation of stigma in schizophrenia using interpretative phenomenological analysis (IPA)'. *Journal of Mental Health* 12 (3), 209-22

206. Lachman, M. E. (1986) 'Locus of Control in Aging Research: A Case for Multidimensional and Domain-Specific Assessment'. *Journal of Psychology and Aging* I (I), 34-40

207. Lafond, R. (2007) 'Reducing seclusion and restraint for improved patient and staff safety'. *Journal of Safe Management of Disruptive and Assaultative Behaviour, September,*8-12, available from: https://www.crisisprevention.com/CPI/media/Media/Blogs/Reducing-Seclusion-and-Restraint-for-Improved-Patient-and-Staff-Safety.pdf

208. Lambert, S. D, and Loiselle, C. G, (2008) 'Combining individual interviews and focus groups to enhance data richness' Journal of Advanced Nursing 62 (2), 228-237

209. Larson, R. (1989) 'Is feeling "in control" related to happiness in daily life?'. *Psychological Reports 64,* 775-784

210. Laugharne, R., Priebe, S., McCabe, R., Garland, N., and Clifford, D. (2011) 'Trust, choice and power in mental health care:

Experiences of patients with psychosis'. *International Journal of Social Psychiatry* 58 (5), 496 –504

211. Leone C, and Burns I. (2000) 'The Measurement of Locus of Control: Assessing More Than Meets *The Eye'. Journal of Psychology*, 134, (1), 63-76
212. Lefcourt, H. M. (1976) *Locus of Control: Current Trends in Theory and Research*. Oxford: Erlbaum.
213. Leff, J. (1990) 'The 'New Cross-Cultural Psychiatry'. A Case of the Baby and the Bathwater'. *The British Journal of Psychiatry: The Journal of Mental Science* 156, 305-307
214. Levenson, H. (1981) 'Differentiating among Internality, Powerful Others, and Chance'. In *Research with the Locus of Control Construct*. ed. by Lefcourt, H. M. New York: Academic Press, 1, 1–15
215. Levenson, H. (1973) 'Multidimensional Locus of Control in Psychiatric Patients'. *Journal of Consulting and Clinical Psychology* 41 (3), 397-404
216. Littlewood, R. (1992) 'Psychiatric Diagnosis and Racial Bias: Empirical and Interpretative Approaches'. *Social Science & Medicine* 34 (2), 141-149
217. Littlewood, R. (1990) 'From Categories to Contexts: A Decade of the "new Cross-Cultural Psychiatry'. *The British Journal of Psychiatry* 156 (3), 308-327
218. Lukes, S. (1974) *Power: A Radical View*. London; New York: Macmillan
219. Lupton, D. (1997) 'Foucault and the Medicalization Critique'. In *Foucault, Health and Medicine*. ed. by Petersen, A. R. and Bunton, R. London: Routledge, 94-110
220. Machery, E. and Faucher, L. (2005) 'Social Construction and the Concept of Race'. *Philosophy of Science* 72 (5), 1208-1219
221. Maden, T. and Spencer-Lane, T. (2010) *Essential Mental Health Law: A Guide to the Revised Mental Health Act and the Mental Capacity Act.* London: Hammersmith press.
222. Mantovani, N., Pizzolati, M., and Edge, D. (2017) 'Exploring the Relationship between Stigma and Help-Seeking for Mental

Illness in African-Descended Faith Communities in the UK'. *Health Expectations: An International Journal of Public Participation in Health Care and Health Policy* 20 (3), 373-384

223. Marshall, G. N. (1991) 'A Multidimensional Analysis of Internal Health Locus of Control Beliefs: Separating the Wheat from the Chaff?'. *Journal of Personality and Social Psychology* 61 (3), 483-491
224. Marshall, G. N., Collins, B. E., and Crooks, V. C. (1990) 'A Comparison of Two Multidimensional Health Locus of Control Instruments'. *Journal of Personality Assessment* 54 (1-2), 181-190
225. Maxwell, J. A. (2005) *Qualitative Research Design: An Interactive Approach*. 2nd edn: Thousand Oaks, CA: SAGE Publications
226. McCabe, R. and Priebe, S. (2004) 'Explanatory models of illness in schizophrenia: comparison of four ethnic groups'. *British Journal of Psychiatry* 185, 25-30
227. McConnell, D. and Gillett, G. (2006) 'Coercion in the therapeutic community'. *Therapeutic Communities* 27, 249–263
228. McKenzie, K., van Os, J., Fahy, T., Jones, P., Harvey, I., Toone, B., and Murray, R. (1995)
229. 'Psychosis with good prognosis in Afro-Caribbean groups now living in the United Kingdom'. *British Medical Journal* 311, 1325-1328
230. McKenzie, K. and Crowcroft, N.S. (1994) 'Race, ethnicity, culture and science'. *British Medical Journal* 309, 286
231. McKenzie, K. and Bhui, K. 2007) 'Institutional racism in mental health care: Services have some way to go before they meet the challenges of a multicultural society'. *BMJ* 334, 649-650
232. Mechanic, D. and Cleary, P. D. (1980) 'Factors associated with the maintenance of positive health behaviour'. *Preventive Medicine* 9, 805-814
233. Meng, M., Xiuwei, Z. and Anli, J. (2011) 'A theoretical framework of caring in the Chinese context: a grounded theory study'. *Journal of Advanced Nursing* 67, 1523–1536

234. Mind (2013) *Mental health crisis care: physical restraint in crisis. A report on physical restraint in hospital settings in England*. Available from: https://www.mind.org.uk/media/197120/physical_restraint_final_web_version.pdf
235. Mind (2017). *Disability discrimination- The Equality Act*, 2010. Available from: https://www.mind.org.uk/media/10520597/disability-discrimination-2017.pdf
236. Mio, J. S. and Iwamasa, J. (1993) 'To Do, or Not to Do: That is the Question for White Cross-Cultural Researchers' *The Counseling Psychologist* 21(2), 197-212
237. Miranda, J., Siddique, S., Belin, T.R., and Kohn-Wood, L.P. (2005) 'Depression prevalence in disadvantaged young black women African and Caribbean immigrants compared to US-born African Americans'. *Soc Psychiatry Psychiatr Epidemiol,* 40 (4), 253–258
238. Mirza, M. (1998) 'Same voices, same lives?': revisiting black feminist standpoint epistemology. In P. Connolly and B. Troyna (eds) Researching Racism in Education: Politics, Theory and Practice. Buckingham: Open University, 79–94
239. Moffat, J., Sass, B., McKenzie, K, and Bhui, K. (2009) 'Improving pathways into mental health care for black and ethnic minority groups: a systematic review of the grey literature'. *Int Rev Psychiatry* 21 (5), 439-49
240. Morgan, C., Mallett, R., Hutchinson, G., Bagalkote, H., Morgan, K., Fearon, P., Dazzan, P., Boydell, J., McKenzie, K., Harrison, G., Murray, R., Jones, P., Craig, T., and Leff, J. (2005) 'Pathways to Care and Ethnicity. 1: Sample Characteristics and Compulsory Admission. Report from the AESOP Study'. *The British Journal of Psychiatry: The Journal of Mental Science* 186, 281-289
241. Morling, B., Kitayama, S. (2008) 'Culture and Motivation'. In *Handbook of Motivation Science*. ed. by Shah J.Y, Gardner, W.L. New York, NY: Guilford Press. 417–433

242. Morrow, M. and Weisser, J. (2012) 'Towards a Social Justice Framework of Mental Health Recovery'. *Studies in Social Justice* 6 (1), 27-43

243. Muhlenkamp, A. F., Brown, N. J., and Sands, D. (1985) 'Determinants of Health Promotion Activities in Nursing Clinic Clients'. *Nursing Research* 34 (6), 327-332

244. Muir-Cochrane, E. (2000) 'The Context of Care: Issues of Power and Control between Patients and Community Mental Health Nurses'. *International Journal of Nursing Practice* 6, 292-299

245. Mulhall, J. (2000) 'Using Community Mental Health Services: Asking Users'. *Practice: Social Work in Action* 12 (4), 27-36

246. Mulholland, H. (2017) *Jacqui Dyer: Talking about Race and Mental Health is Everyone's Business | Hélène Mulholland* [online] available from <http://www.theguardian.com/society/2017/nov/08/jacqui-dyer-race-mental-health-act-black-people-detentions-inequality>

247. Mulveen, R. and Hepworth, J. (2006) 'An Interpretative Phenomenological Analysis of Participation in a Pro-Anorexia Internet Site and its Relationship with Disordered Eating'. *Journal of Health Psychology* 11 (2), 283-296

248. National Health Services (2017) *Mental Health Act Statistics, Annual Figures: 2016-17.* Available from: https://digital.nhs.uk/.../Mental-Health...Statistics.../ment-heal-act-stat-eng-2016-17-sum-rep.pdf

249. National Health Services (2016) *The Five Year Forward View for Mental Health: A Report from the Independent Mental Health Taskforce to the NHS in England.* Available from: www.england.nhs.uk/wp-content/uploads/2016/02/Mental-Health-Taskforce-FYFV-final.pdf

250. *National Health Services, South West London Collaborative Commissioning (2014) South West London 5 Year Strategic Plan.* Available from: http://www.swlccgs.nhs.uk/wp-content/uploads/2014/06/SWL-5-year-strategic-plan.pdf

251. National Health Services (2013) *The Six Caldicott Principles.* Available from: www.connectingforhealth.nhs.uk/systemsandservices/infogov/caldicott

252. National Health Services, N. (2016) *Implementing the Five Year Forward View for Mental Health.* Available from: www.england.nhs.uk/wp-content/uploads/2016/07/fyfv-mh.pdf

253. National Institute for Mental Health in England (2008) *Report of the Community Led Research Project Focussing on Male African and African Caribbean Perspectives on Recovery.* Available from: https://recoverydevon.co.uk/mdocs-posts/afro-caribbean-perspectives-2008/

254. Newton-Howes, G. and Mullen, R, (2011) 'Coercion in psychiatric care: systematic review of correlates and topics'. *Psychiatr Serv*, 62 (5), 465-70

255. Ng, T. W. H., Sorensen, K. L., and Eby, L. T. (2006) 'Locus of control at work: A meta-analysis'.

256. *Journal of Organizational Behavior* 27, 1057– 1087

257. Nguyen, T. (2015) 'The Interconnection between Interpretivist Paradigm and Qualitative Methods in Education'. *American Journal of Educational Science* 1 (2), 24-27

258. Nicholson, R, A., Ekenstam, C., and Norwood, S. (1996) 'Coercion and the Outcome of Psychiatric Hospitalization'. *International Journal of Law and Psychiatry* 19 (2), 201-217

259. Norfolk, Suffolk and Cambridgeshire Strategic Health Authority (2003). *Independent inquiry into the death of David Bennett.* Available from: www.irr.org.uk/pdf/bennett_inquiry.pdf

260. Norman, P., Bennett, P., Smith, C., and Murphy, S. (1998) 'Health Locus of Control and Health Behaviour'. *Journal of Health Psychology* 3, 170-180

261. Ogunyemi, K. (2013) 'Ethics education and locus of control: Is Rotter's scale valid for Nigeria?'. *African Journal of Business Ethics* 7 (1), 1-10

262. O'Brien, A. J. and Golding, C.G. (2003) 'Coercion in mental healthcare: the principle of leastcoercive care'. *Journal of Psychiatric and Mental Health Nursing* 10: 167–173

263. Office of National Statistics (2014) *Population Estimates by Ethnic Group (PEEGs).* Available from: http://www.ons.gov.uk/ons/search/index.html?pageSize=50&sortBy=none&sortDirection=none&newquery=black+population+in+wandsworth

264. O'Leary, K. D. and Drabman, R. S. (1971) 'Token reinforcement programs in the classroom: A Review'. *Psychological Bulletin* 75, 379-398

265. Palinkas, L. A., Horwitz, S.M., Green, C.A., Wisdom, J.P., Duan, N., and Hoagwood, K. (2015) 'Purposeful Sampling for Qualitative Data Collection and Analysis in Mixed Method Implementation Research'. *Adm Policy Ment Health* 42, 533–544

266. Palys, T. (2008) Purposive sampling. In *The Sage Encyclopedia of Qualitative Research Methods. (Vol.2).* ed. by Given, L.M. Los Angeles: Sage. pp. 697-8.

267. Papadakis, M. and Carolissen, R. (2012) 'Deconstructing the focus group as a transformative methodology and potential intervention'. *International Journal of Psychology* (47) (sup1), 666-672

268. Papadopoulos, C. (2009). *Stigma towards groups with mental health problems: an individualism-collectivism cross-cultural comparison.* [Online] thesis or dissertation. Available from EThOS – Electronic Theses Online Service

269. Parton, N. (2003) 'Rethinking Professional Practice: The contributions of Social Constructionism and the Feminist 'Ethics of Care''. *British Journal of Social Work* 33, 1-16

270. Pease, B. (2002) 'Rethinking Empowerment: A Postmodern Reappraisal for Emancipatory Practice'. *The British Journal of Social Work* 32 (2), 135-147

271. Peterson, C. and Stunkard, A. J. (1989) 'Personal Control and Health Promotion'. *Social Science & Medicine (1982)* 28 (8), 819-828

272. Ponto, M. T. (2004) *Locus of Control, an Exploration of the Nursing Students' Views on Control, Autonomy and Satisfaction.* [Online] thesis or dissertation. Available from: EThOS – Electronic Theses Online Service

273. Prince, M., Stewart, R., Ford, T. &Hoptopf, M. (2003) *Practical Psychiatric Epidemiology*. Oxford, New York: Oxford University Press

274. Proto, E., & Quintana-Domeque, C. (2020). COVID-19 and Mental Health Deterioration among BAME Groups in the UK. Available at: https://www.cesifo.org/en/publikationen/2020/working-paper/covid-19-and-mental-health-deterioration-among-bame-groups-uk

275. Rahman, M. S. (2016) 'The Advantages and Disadvantages of using Qualitative and Quantitative Approaches and Methods in Language "Testing and Assessment" Research: A Literature Review'. *Journal of Education and Learning* 6 (1), 102-112

276. Rathwell, T. and Phillips, D. (1987) *'Health Race and Ethnicity'*. UK: Croom Help Ltd.

277. Rauckhorst, L. M. (1987) 'Health Habits of Elderly Widows'. *Journal of Gerontological Nursing* 13 (8), 19-22

278. Redsell, S. A. and Cheater, F. M. (2001) 'The Data Protection Act (1998): Implications for Health Researchers'. *Journal of Advanced Nursing* 35 (4), 508-513

279. Roach, S. (1987) *The Human Act of Caring* Ottawa: The Canadian Hospital Association Available from <https://www.goodreads.com/book/show/6850787-the-human-act-of-caring>

280. Robinson, M., Keating, F., and Robertson, S. (2011) ''Ethnicity, Gender and Mental Health'.

281. *Diversity in Health and Care* 8, 81-92

282. Rotter, J. B. (1966) 'Generalized Expectancies for Internal Versus External Control of Reinforcement' *Psychological Monographs: General and Applied* 80: 1–28 [online] available from <http://dx.doi.org/10.1037/h0092976> []

283. Ruggiero, K. M. and Taylor, D. M. (1997) 'Why Minority Group Members Perceive Or do Not Perceive the Discrimination that Confronts them: The Role of Self-Esteem and Perceived Control'. *Journal of Personality and Social Psychology* 72 (2), 373-389

284. Ruiz-Casares, M. (2014) 'Mental Health: Tailor Informed-Consent Processes'. *Nature* 513 (7518), 304

285. Rutter, D., Francis, J., Coren, E., Fisher, M. (2010) *SCIE Systematic Research Reviews: Guidelines (2nd Edition)*. Social Care Institute for Excellence. Available at: http://www.scie.org.uk/publications/researchresources/rr01.pdf

286. Saltzer, E. B. (1982) 'The Weight Locus of Control (WLOC) Scale: A Specific Measure for Obesity Research'. *Journal of Personality Assessment* 46, 620-628

287. Santiago, J. H. and Tarantino, S J. (2002) 'Individualism and Collectivism: Cultural Orientation in Locus of Control and Moral Attribution under Conditions of Change'. *Psychological Reports* 91, 1168.

288. Sarup, M. (1993) 'Foucault and the Social Sciences'. In *An Introductory Guide to Post-Structuralism and Post-Modernism.* ed. by Sarup, M. Harlow: Longman, 58-89

289. Sashidharan, S. P. (2001) 'Institutional Racism in British Psychiatry'. *Psychiatric Bulletin* 25, 244-247

290. Schneider, B, Ali, J, Arney, L, Benson, G, Calderbank, C, Mathieu, C, Misurelli, M, Mitchell, M, Silbernagel, D, Sunderland, M (2010) *Housing for Groups Living with Schizophrenia: Dilemmas of Care and Control.* University of Calgary

291. Schram, T. H. (2003) *Conceptualizing Qualitative Inquiry.* Upper Saddle River, NJ: Merrill. Prentice Hall.

292. Schuh, S, Hernandez, B. A, Van Quaquebeke, N, Hossiep, R, Frieg, P, Dick, R (2014) 'Gender Differences in Leadership Role Occupancy: The Mediating Role of Power Motivation'. *Journal of Business Ethics* 120 (3), 363-379

293. Scotland, J. (2012) 'Exploring the Philosophical Underpinnings of Research: Relating Ontology and Epistemology to the Methodology and Methods of the Scientific, Interpretive, and Critical Research Paradigms'. *English Language Teaching* 5 (9), 9-16

294. Seebohm, P, Chaudhary, S, Boyce, M, Elkan, R, Avis, M, Munn-Giddings, C (2013)) 'The Contribution of Self-Help/Mutual Aid Groups to Mental Well-being Health and Social Care in the Community'. *Health and Social Care in the Community* 21 (4), 391-401

295. Seeman, M. and Seeman, T. E (1983) 'Health Behaviour and Personal Autonomy: A Longitudinal Study of the Sense of Control in Illness'. *Journal of Health and Social Behaviour* 24, 144-160

296. Sengul, Y., Kara, B., and Arda, M (2010) 'The Relationship between Health Locus of Control and Quality of Life in Patients with Chronic Back Pain'. *Turkish Neurosurgery* 20, 180-185

297. Sewell, H. (2008) *Working with Ethnicity, Race and Culture in Mental Health: A Handbook for Practitioners*. London: Jessica Kingsley Publishers

298. Sigurvinsdotti, R., Thorisdottir, I.E., &Gylfason, H.F. (2020). The Impact of COVID-19 on Mental Health: The Role of Locus on Control and Internet Use. *Int. J. Environ. Res. Public Health.*; 17,(6985), 1-15

299. Slivinske, L. R. and Fitch, V. L (1987) 'The Effects of Control-Enhancing Interventions on the Well-being of Elderly Individuals Living in Retirement Communities'. *The Gerontologist* 27, 176-181

300. Smith, G.M., Altenor, A.A., and Davies, R. H (2006) 'In Reply: Elimination of Seclusion and Restraint: A Reasonable Goal?'. *Psychiatric Services* 57 (4), 576-581

301. Smith, J. (2004) 'Reflecting on the Development of Interpretative Phenomenological Analysis and its Contribution to Qualitative Research in Psychology'. *Qualitative Research in Psychology* 1, 39-54

302. Smith, J.A., Flowers, P., Larkin, M (2012) *Interpretative Phenomenological Analysis: Theory, Method and Research*. London: Sage.

303. Smith K., Bhui K., &Cipriani A. (2020). COVID-19, mental health and ethnic minorities. *Evidence-Based Mental Health*. 23, (3), 89–90.

304. Smyth, G., Harries, P., and Dorer, G. (2011) 'Exploring Mental Health Service Users' Experiences of Social Inclusion in their Community Occupations'. *The British Journal of Occupational Therapy* 74 (7), 323-331

305. Sørgaard, K. W. (2007) 'Satisfaction and Coercion among Voluntary, Persuaded/Pressured and Committed Patients in Acute Psychiatric Treatment'. *Scandinavian Journal of Caring Sciences* 21 (2), 214-219

306. Sørgaard, K. W. (2004) 'Patients' Perception of Coercion in Acute Psychiatric Wards. an Intervention Study'. *Nordic Journal of Psychiatry* 58 (4), 299-304

307. Starks, H. and Trinidad, S. B. (2007) 'Choose Your Method: A Comparison of Phenomenology, Discourse Analysis, and Grounded Theory'. *Qualitative Health Research* 17 (10), 1372-1380

308. Steptoe, A., Wardle, J., Vinck, J., Tuomisto, M., Holte, A., and Wichstrøm, L. (1994) 'Personality and Attitudinal Correlates of Healthy and Unhealthy Lifestyles in Young Adults'. *Psychology & Health* 9 (5), 331-343

309. Stewart, D.W. &Shamdasami, P. N. (1990) *Focus Groups: Theory and Practice*. London: Sage.

310. Strickland, B. R. (1978) 'Internal-External Expectancies and Health-Related Behaviors'. *Journal of Consulting and Clinical Psychology* 46 (6), 1192-1211

311. Suizzo, M. and Soon, K. (2006) 'Parental Academic Socialization: Effects of Home-Based Parental Involvement on Locus of Control across U.S. Ethnic Groups'. *Educational Psychology* 26 (6), 827-846
312. Sullivan, P. (1998) 'Care and Control in Mental Health Nursing'. *Nursing Standard* 13 (15), 42-45
313. Takizawa, R., Maughan, B., and Arseneault, L. (2014) 'Adult Health Outcomes of Childhood Bullying Victimization: Evidence from a Five-Decade Longitudinal British Birth Cohort'. *The American Journal of Psychiatry* 171 (7), 777-784
314. Taylor, B., Kermode, S., and Roberts, K. (2007) *Research in Nursing and Health Care: Evidence for Practice*. Sydney: Thomson.
315. Taylor, S. E., Lichtman, R. R., and Wood, J. V. (1984) 'Attributions, Beliefs about Control, and Adjustment to Breast Cancer'. *Journal of Personality and Social Psychology* 46 (3), 489-502
316. Taylor, S. E. (1979) 'Hospital Patient Behavior: Reactance, Helplessness, Or Control?'. *Journal of Social Issues* 35 (1), 156-184
317. Teijlingen, E V. and Hundley, V. (2002) 'The importance of pilot studies'. *Nursing Standard.* 16 (40), 33-36
318. Thabane, L., Ma, J., Chu, R., Cheng, J., Ismaila, A., Rios, L. P., Robson, R., Thabane, M., Giangregorio, L., and Goldsmith, C. H. (2010) 'A Tutorial on Pilot Studies: The what, Why and How'. *BMC Medical Research Methodology* 10, 1 Available at: https://doi.org/10.1186/1471-2288-10-1
319. Thanh, N. C, Thanh, T. T. L (2015) 'the Interconnection between Interpretivist Paradigm and Qualitative Methods in Education'. *American Journal of Educational Science* 1 (2), 24-27
320. Thomas, P. Y. (2010) *Towards Developing a Web-Based Blended Learning Environment at the University of Botswana.* [Online] thesis or dissertation. Available from: http://uir.unisa.ac.za/handle/10500/4245?show=full.

321. Thompson, S. C. (1981) 'A Complex Answer to a Simple Question: Will it Hurt Less if I can Control it?'. *Psychological Bulletin* 90, 89-101

322. Tigani, X., Artemiadis, A. K., Alexopoulos, E. C., Chrousos, G. P., and Darviri, C. (2011) 'Gender Differences in Greek Centenarians. A Cross-Sectional Nation-Wide Study, Examining Multiple Socio-Demographic and Personality Factors and Health Locus of Control'. *BMC Geriatrics* 11 (87), 1-8

323. Timmers, G. J., Schouten, J. A., ter Wee, P. M., and Gans, R. O. (1999) 'Hypertension in the Negro Patient'. *Nederlands Tijdschrift Voor Geneeskunde* 143 (5), 229-234

324. Tobin, S. J. and Raymundo, M. M. (2010) 'Causal Uncertainty and Psychological Well-being: The Moderating Role of Accommodation (Secondary Control)'. *Personality & Social Psychology Bulletin* 36 (3), 371-383

325. Tokuda, Y., Takahashi, O., Ohde, S., Ogata, H., Yanai, H., Shimbo, T., Fukuhara, S., Hinohara, S., Fukui, T. (2007) 'Health Locus of Control and use of Conventional and Alternative Care'. *The British Journal of General Practice* 57 (541), 643-649

326. Torelli, C. J. and Shavitt, S. (2010) 'Culture and Concepts of Power'. *Journal of Personality and Social Psychology* 99 (4), 703-723

327. Torrey, E. F. and Zdanowicz, M. (2001) 'Outpatient Commitment: What, Why, and for Whom'. *Psychiatric Services (Washington, D.C.)* 52 (3), 337-341

328. Treacy, S., Reidy, H., Webber, M. (2015) *Evaluation of the Croydon Reablement Service*: University of York. Available at: https://www.york.ac.uk/media/spsw/documents/cmhsr/CroydonReablementEvaluation2015.pdf

329. Triandis, H. C. (1995a) *Individualism and Collectivism.* CO: Westview: Boulder,

330. Triandis, H. C. (1995b) Motivation and achievement in collectivist and individualist cultures. In. *Advances in motivation and achievement. E*d. by Maehr, M. L. Pintrich, P. R. Greenwich, CT: JAI, 1–30

331. Triandis, H. C. and Suh, E. M. (2002) 'Cultural Influences on Personality'. *Annual Review of Psychology* 53, 133-160
332. Triandis, H. C. (2001) 'Individualism and Collectivism: Past, Present, and Future'. In *The Handbook of Culture and Psychology*. ed. by Matsumoto, D. New York: Oxford University, 35-50
333. Trivedi, P. and Wykes, T. (2002) 'From Passive Subjects to Equal Partners: Qualitative Review of User Involvement in Research'. *The British Journal of Psychiatry: The Journal of Mental Science* 181, 468-472
334. Verkerk, M. A. (2001) 'The Care Perspective and Autonomy'. *Medicine, Health Care, and Philosophy* 4 (3), 289-294
335. Wainwright, S. P. and Forbes, A. (2000) 'Philosophical Problems with Social Research on Health Inequalities'. *Health Care Analysis: HCA: Journal of Health Philosophy and Policy* 8 (3), 259-277
336. Wall, S, Churchill, R, Hotopf, M. Buchanan, A, Simon Wessely (1) (1999) *A Systematic Review of Research Relating to the Mental Health Act (1983)*. London: Department of Health
337. Waller, K. V. and Bates, R. C. (1992) 'Health Locus of Control and Self-Efficacy Beliefs in a Healthy Elderly Sample'. *American Journal of Health Promotion: AJHP* 6 (4), 302-309
338. Wallston, B. D. and Wallston, K. A. (1978) 'Locus of Control and Health: A Review of the Literature'. *Health Education Monographs* 6 (2), 107-117
339. Wallston, B. S., Wallston, K. A., Kaplan, G. D., and Maides, S. A. (1976) 'Development and Validation of the Health Locus of Control (HLC) Scale'. *Journal of Consulting and Clinical Psychology* 44 (4), 580-585
340. Wallston, K. A., Wallston, B. S., and DeVellis, R. (1978) 'Development of the Multidimensional Health Locus of Control (MHLC) Scales'. *Health Education Monographs* 6 (2), 160-170
341. Wallston, K. A., & Wallston, B. S (1980) 'Health Locus of Control Scales'. In *Advances and Innovations in Locus of Control*

Research. ed. by Lefcourt, H. New York: Academic Press., 198-234

342. Wallston, K. A., & Wallston, B. S. (1981) 'Health Locus of Control Scales'. In *Research with the Locus of Control Construct*. ed. by Lefcourt, H. New York: Academic Press., 1, 189-243
343. Wallston, K. A., Wallston, B. S. (1982) 'Who is Responsible for Your Health? The Construct of Health Locus of Control'. In *Social Psychology of Health and Illness*. ed. by Sanders, G, Suls, J. Hillsdale, NJ: Erlbaum., 65-95
344. Wallston, K. A. (1992) 'Hocus-Pocus, the Focus Isn't Strictly on Locus: Rotter's Social Learning Theory Modified for Health'. *Cognitive Therapy and Research* 16 (2), 183-199
345. Wang, D., Wang, Y., Zhang, Y. (1992) 'The Relationship between Locus of Control, Depression, Shame, and Self-Esteem'. *Chinese Mental Health Journal* 6, 207-210
346. Watson, J. (2008) *Nursing: The Philosophy and Science of Caring*. Revised Edition edn. Colorado: The University Press of Colorado
347. Watson, J. (1979) 'Nursing: The Philosophy and Science of Caring'. *Nursing Administration Quarterly* 3 (4), 86-87
348. Weaver, K. and Olson, J. K. (2006) 'Understanding Paradigms used for Nursing Research'. *Journal of Advanced Nursing* 53 (4), 459-469
349. Weiss, G. L. and Larsen, D. L. (1990) 'Health Value, Health Locus of Control, and the Prediction of Health Protective Behaviors'. *Social Behavior and Personality* 18 (1), 121-136
350. Weisz, J. R., Eastman, K. L., and McCarty, C. A. (1996) 'Primary and Secondary Control in East Asia: Comments on Oerter Et Al'. *Culture & Psychology* 2 (1), 63-76
351. Williams, A., Katz, L (2001) 'The use of Focus Group Methodology in Education: Some Theoretical and Practical Considerations'. *International Electronic Journal for Leadership in Learning* 5 (3), 1-10
352. Williams, J, Keating, F. (2005) '10 Social Inequalities and Mental Health: An Integrative Approach'. In *Beyond the Water Towers:*

The Unfinished Revolution in Mental Health Services 1985-2005. ed. by Bell, A. London: Sainsbury Centre for Mental Health

353. Williams, S., Wilson, A., Myrie, L., Collymore, M. (2006) *Report of the Community-Led Research Project Focusing on the Mental Health Service Needs of African and African Caribbean Women.* Available at: http://www.lemosandcrane.co.uk/bluesalmon/resources/DoH%20-%20Report%20of%20the%20community-led%20research%20project%20focusing%20on%20the%20mental%20health%20service%20needs%20of%20African%20and%20African%20Caribbean%20women.pdf
354. Williamson, R., Lauricella, K., Browning, A., Tierney, E., Chen, J., Joseph, S., Sharrock, J., Trauer, T., and Hamilton, B. (2014) 'Patient Factors Associated with Incidents of Aggression in a General Inpatient Setting'. *Journal of Clinical Nursing* 23 (7-8), 1144-1152
355. Willig, C. (2003) *Introducing Qualitative Research in Psychology: Adventures in Theory and Method.* Open University Press.
356. Wilson, M. (2011) *Delivering Race Equality Action Plan: A Five Year Review.* Department of Health. Available at: www.hsconsultancy.org.uk/system/resources/1/race-equality-action-plan-a-five-year-review.pdf?1302161027
357. Wiseman, V. (1997) 'Caring: The Neglected Health Outcome? Or Input?'. *Health Policy (Amsterdam, Netherlands)* 39 (1), 43-53
358. Wood, W. D. and Letak, J. K. (1982) 'A Mental-Health Locus of Control Scale'. *Personality and Individual Differences* 3 (1), 84-87
359. Yardley, L., Bishop, F. (2015) 'Using Mixed Methods in Health Research: Benefits and Challenges'. *British Journal of Health Psychology* 20, 1-4

Printed in Great Britain
by Amazon

63242737R00189